ETHICAL PRACTICES IN SPEECH-LANGUAGE PATHOLOGY AND AUDIOLOGY

CASE STUDIES

ETHICAL PRACTICES IN SPEECH-LANGUAGE PATHOLOGY AND AUDIOLOGY

CASE STUDIES

MARY PANNBACKER, PH.D.
Professor and Program Director
Department of Communication Disorders
Louisiana State University Medical Center
Shreveport, Louisiana

GRACE F. MIDDLETON, ED.D.
Professor
Program in Speech-Language Pathology
College of Nursing and Health Sciences
University of Texas at El Paso

GAY T. VEKOVIUS, M.S.
Assistant Professor
Department of Communication Disorders
Louisiana State University Medical Center
Shreveport, Louisiana

SINGULAR PUBLISHING GROUP, INC.
SAN DIEGO · LONDON

Singular Publishing Group, Inc.
4284 41st Street
San Diego, California 92105–1197

19 Compton Terrace
London, N1 2UN, UK

Typeset in 10/12 Times by So Cal Graphics
Printed in the United States of America by McNaughton & Gunn

Library of Congress Cataloging-in-Publication Data

Pannbacker, Mary H.
    Ethical practices in speech-language pathology and audiology:
  case studies / Mary Pannbacker, Grace F. Middleton, Gay T. Vekovius.
     p.   cm.
    Includes bibliographical references and index.
    ISBN 1-56593-280-3
    1. Speech therapists—Professional ethics. 2. Audiologists—
  Professional ethics. I. Middleton, Grace. II. Vekovius, Gay T.
  III. Title.
  RC428.5.P36   1995
  174'.2—dc20
                                      95-34209
                                         CIP

CONTENTS

TABLES

FIGURES

FOREWORD

Ethics, as a branch of philosophy, is a discipline of long-standing history. As a social imperative, however, it has gained stature much more recently owing largely to public reaction to a few instances, albeit sensational ones, of professional misconduct. As a result, some codes of professional conduct have been lifted from dusty shelves and given new, more exciting covers. In other instances, codes have been developed where they had not previously existed. The value of professional codes of conduct is not so much that they exist but rather that they are practiced. It is in the daily practice of the profession (in the fullest sense of that phrase) that one must find the vitality of ethical conduct. That is what this book is all about.

Through a series of well-defined and practical case studies, the reader is presented with the kinds of ethical dilemmas that confront audiologists and speech-language pathologists in the day-to-day practice of their professions. The case studies cover a broad spectrum of contexts and circumstances—literally, something for everyone— in which critical variables are used to guide one through the ethical decision-making process. After all, that is what ethical conduct is all about. It is about real circumstances, conflicting interests, and the challenge of developing resolutions based on principles and values that rise above self-interest.

There is nothing easy about making ethical decisions. The dilemmas we confront do not come packaged with ready answers. Rather, they tend to be a collection of unique circumstances—at least unique to our own experiences— and we must find our own way in resolving them. Codes of ethics cannot give us the resolutions. They can direct us, but we must search for answers on our own. Ethical decision making is ultimately a lonely process in that regard. But there are signposts and pathways to help us along. You will find many of them on the pages that follow. Happy journey.

Joseph W. Helmick, Ph.D.
Dean of Graduate Studies and Research
Texas Christian University
Fort Worth, Texas

PREFACE

Ethics are an important part of speech-language pathology and audiology, although many students are not adequately prepared about ethics. Resnick (1993) indicated that "some schools provide courses for students enrolled in professional programs, but they are largely elective offerings and the formal teaching of professional ethics remains underemphasized" (p. 148). The typical method of providing information to students about the American Speech-Language-Hearing Association's (ASHA) Code of Ethics by providing them with a copy of the code and encouraging them to adhere to these principles does not help students realize the importance of ethical professional conduct (Gonzalez & Coleman, 1994; Seymour, 1994).

The teaching of ethics and the process of ethical decision making have received more attention in dentistry, medicine, nursing and occupational therapy than in speech-language pathology and audiology (Ales, Charlson, Williams-Russo, & Allegrante, 1992; Babapulle, 1992; Baylis & Downie, 1991; Bebeau, Rest, & Yamoor, 1985; Bickel, 1991; Burling et al., 1990; Cohen, Singer, Rothman, & Robb, 1991; DeMars, Fleming, & Benham, 1991; Dickstein, Erlen, & Erlen, 1991; Feudtner, Christakis, & Christakis, 1994; Hundert, 1987; Jonsen, 1990; Kalichman & Friedman, 1992; Ledbetter, 1991; Macrina & Munro, 1993; Miles, Lane, Bickel, Walker, & Cassel, 1989; Mitchell, Lovat & Myser, 1992; Mustapha & Seybert, 1989; O'Neil, 1991; Rezler et al., 1992; Ryden, Duckett, Crisham, Caplan, & Schmitz, 1989; Sachs & Siegler, 1993; Seedhouse, 1991; Strong, Beckmann, & Dacus, 1992; Strong, Connelly, & Forrow, 1992; Turner & Rufo, 1992; Waithe, Duckett, Schmitz, Crisham, & Ryden, 1989; White, Hickson, Theriot, & Zaner, 1991).

The importance of ethics instruction in speech-language pathology and audiology has recently received attention. Seymour (1990) suggested that "as professionals it is our responsibility to educate and prepare our students to think about relevant ethical issues by way of curriculum offerings in order to protect the special needs of our patients, clients and consumers" (p. 93). Waggoner (1992–1993) indicated "the teaching of ethics is critically needed in undergraduate and professional school curricula" (p. 114). Pannbacker,

Middleton, and Lass (1994) believe ethics should be included in the training of speech-language pathologists and audiologists. ASHA (1994a) stated "understanding ethical canons is the joint responsibility of the individual and of our educational institutions . . . principles of ethics can and must be taught with the very same rigor that we would use to teach scientific method" (p. 18).

Many practicing speech-language pathologists and audiologists have had little formal training in ethics and ethical decision making. Often such training in these areas has been informal and does not go beyond role modeling. This type of training may be less than satisfactory. Furthermore, the increasing complexity of ethical issues in health care underscores the need for continuing education about ethics and ethical decision making (Pannbacker, Lass, & Middleton, 1993). Technological advances, the development of interprofessional health care teams, the increasingly multipolitical nature of society, and the patients' rights movement require increasingly complex decision making. Furthermore, the increased emphasis on the legal and ethical responsibilities of speech-language pathologists and audiologists supports the need for training in ethical decision making as well as decision implementation (ASHA, 1994b; Silverman, 1992).

There are several strategies that can be used to provide information about ethics and ethical decision making. Case studies and the need to emphasize dilemma discussion in teaching ethics have been suggested (ASHA, 1994c; Reichert & Caruso, 1990–1991; Seymour, 1994). Gonzalez and Coleman (1994) reported that students prefer the case study approach to ethics education because it provides a broader understanding of professional issues, assists in problem solving, and has applicability to real clinical situations. Waggoner (1992–1993) described the use of computer simulation models. Other strategies for teaching ethics include surveys, outside assignment formats, and the traditional lecture (Gonzalez & Coleman, 1994; Seymour, 1994).

Information about professional ethics in speech-language pathology and audiology is primarily related to clinical practicum. Ethical issues related to research have received less attention and academic issues have received almost no attention.

This book is for anyone interested in ethics in speech-language pathology and audiology. It is about ethical issues related to academia, clinical practice, and research. The purposes of this book are threefold: (1) to provide an overview of ethics related to speech-language pathology and audiology, (2) to provide for practical application of ethics related to professional issues, and (3) to describe available resource materials related to ethical issues in speech-language pathology and audiology.

This book is divided into five chapters. The first chapter provides an overview of ethics in speech-language pathology and audiology. The case studies are organized into three chapters: academic, clinical, and research. Each case study is composed of background information, the areas of

ASHA's and the American Academy of Audiology's (AAA) Codes of Ethics that might apply, possible solutions, discussion questions, and references. The case studies are based on simulated situations and actual experience(s). Readers are encouraged to propose additional solutions.

The fifth chapter is a list of resource materials on ethical issues. The book contains the Code of Ethics of the American Speech-Language-Hearing Association (Appendix C), the Code of Ethics of the American Academy of Audiology (Appendix D), and a glossary of ethical terms.

REFERENCES

Ales, K. L., Charlson, M. E., Williams-Russo, P., & Allegrante, J. P. (1992). Using faculty consensus to develop and implement a medical ethics course. *Academic Medicine, 67*(6), 406–408.

American Speech-Language-Hearing Association. (1994a). Ethics in research and professional practice. *Asha, 36* (Suppl. 13), 17–18.

American Speech-Language-Hearing Association. (1994b). Professional liability and risk management for the audiology and speech-language pathology professions. *Asha, 36* (Suppl. 12), 25–38.

American Speech-Language-Hearing Association. (1994c). *Ethics education kit*. Rockville, MD: Author.

Babapulle, C. J. (1992). Teaching of medical ethics in Sri Lanka. *Medical Education, 26*, 185–189.

Baylis, F., & Downie, J. (1991). Ethics education for Canadian medical students. *Academic Medicine, 66*(7), 413–414.

Bebeau, M. J., Rest, J. R., & Yamoor, C. M. (1985). Measuring dental students' ethical sensitivity. *Journal of Dental Education, 49*(4), 225–235.

Bickel, J. (1991). Medical students' professional ethics: Defining the problems and developing resources. *Academic Medicine, 66*(12), 726–729.

Burling, S. J., Lumley, J. S. P., McCarthy, L. S. L., Mytton, J. A., Nolan, J. A., Sissou, P., Williams, D. G., & Wright, L. J. (1990). Review of the teaching of medical ethics in London medical schools. *Journal of Medical Ethics, 16*, 206–209.

Cohen, R., Singer, P. A., Rothman, A. I., & Robb, A. (1991). Assessing competency to address ethical issues in medicine. *Academic Medicine, 66*(1), 14–15.

DeMars, P. A., Fleming, J. D., & Benham, P. A. (1991). Ethics across the occupational therapy curriculum. *American Journal of Occupational Therapy, 45*(9), 782–787.

Dickstein, E., Erlen, J., & Erlen, J. A. (1991). Ethical principles contained in currently professed medical oaths. *Academic Medicine, 66*(10), 622–624.

Feudtner, C., Christakis, D. A., & Christakis, N. A. (1994). Do clinical clerks suffer ethical erosion? Students' perceptions of their ethical environment and personal development. *Academic Medicine, 69*(8), 670–679.

Gonzalez, L. S., & Coleman, R. O. (1994). Ethics education: Students prefer case study approach. *Asha, 36*(8), 47–48.

Hundert, E. M. (1987). A model for ethical problem solving in medicine, with practical applications. *American Journal of Psychiatry, 144*(7), 839–846.

Jonsen, A. R. (1990). *The new medicine and the old ethics.* Cambridge, MA: Harvard University Press.

Kalichman, M. W., & Friedman, P. J. (1992). A pilot study of biomedical trainees' perceptions concerning research ethics. *Academic Medicine, 67*(11), 769–775.

Ledbetter, E. O. (1991). Ethics education in medicine. *Advances in Pediatrics, 38*, 365–386.

Macrina, F. L., & Munro, C. L. (1993). Graduate training in principles of scientific integrity. *Academic Medicine, 68*(12), 879–884.

Miles, S., Lane, L., Bickel, J., Walker, R., & Cassel, C. (1989). Medical ethics education is coming of age. *Academic Medicine, 64*, 705–714.

Mitchell, K. R., Lovat, T. J., & Myser, C. M. (1992). Teaching bioethics to medical students: The Newcastle experience. *Medical Education, 26*, 290–300.

Mustapha, S., & Seybert, J. (1989). Moral reasoning in college students: Implications for nursing education. *Journal of Nursing Education, 28*(3), 107–111.

O'Neil, J. A. (1991). Teaching basic ethical concepts and decision making: A staff development application. *Journal of Continuing Education in Nursing, 22*(5), 184–188.

Pannbacker, M. H., Lass, N. J., & Middleton, G. F. (1993). Ethics education in speech-language pathology and audiology training programs. *Asha, 35*(4), 53–55.

Pannbacker, M. H., Middleton, G. F., & Lass, N. J. (1994). Ethics education for speech-language pathologists and audiologists. *Asha, 36*(9), 40–43.

Reichert, A. M., & Caruso, A. J. (1990–1991). Ethical standards in the university clinic: A student perspective. *National Student Speech Language Hearing Association, 18*, 137–141.

Resnick, D. M. (1993). *Professional ethics for speech-language pathologists and audiologists.* San Diego: Singular Publishing.

Rezler A. C., Schwartz, R. L., Obenshain, S. S., Lambert, P., Gibson, J., & Bennchum, D. A. (1992). Assessment of ethical decisions and values. *Medical Education, 26*, 7–16.

Ryden, M. B., Duckett, L., Crisham, P., Caplan, A., & Schmitz, K. (1989). Multi-course sequential learning as a model for content integration: Ethics as a prototype. *Journal of Nursing Education, 28*(3), 102–106.

Sachs, G. A., & Siegler, M. (1993). Teaching scientific integrity and the responsible conduct of research. *Academic Medicine, 68*(12), 871–875.

Seedhouse, D. F. (1991). Health care ethics teaching for medical students. *Medical Education, 25,* 230–237.

Seymour, C. M. (1990). The hunt for absolute goodness. In American Speech-Language-Hearing Association. *Reflections on ethics* (pp. 91–93). Rockville, MD: American Speech-Language-Hearing Association.

Seymour, C. M. (1994). Ethical considerations. In R. Lubinski & C. Frattali (Eds.), *Professional issues in speech-language pathology and audiology* (pp. 61–74). San Diego: Singular Publishing Group.

Silverman, F. H. (1992). *Legal-ethical considerations, restrictions, and obligations for clinicians who treat communication disorders.* Springfield, IL: Charles C. Thomas Publishers.

Strong, C., Beckmann, C. R. B., & Dacus, J. V. (1992). A conference on ethics for obstetric and gynecological clerkship students. *Medical Education, 26,* 354–359.

Strong, C., Connelly, J. E., & Forrow, L. (1992). Teachers' perceptions of difficulties in teaching ethics in residencies. *Academic Medicine, 67*(6), 398–402.

Turner, S. L., & Rufo, M. K. (1992). An overview of nursing ethics for nurse educators. *Journal of Continuing Education in Nursing, 23*(6), 272–277.

Waggoner, K. M. (1992–1993). Teaching professional ethics. *National Student Speech-Language-Hearing Association Journal, 20,* 112–121.

Waithe, M. E., Duckett, L., Schmitz, K., Crisham, P., & Ryden, M. (1989). Developing case situations for ethics education in nursing. *Journal of Nursing Education, 28,* 175–180.

White, B. D., Hickson, G. B., Theriot, R., & Zaner, R. M. (1991). A medical ethics issues survey of residents in five pediatric training programs. *American Journal of Diseases of Children, 145,* 161–164.

ACKNOWLEDGMENTS

There are many people to whom we owe our thanks. Especially acknowledged are those students and colleagues who have taught us about ethics. The valuable help of librarians at Louisiana State University Medical Center is acknowledged. Those were: Kerri Christopher, David Duggan, and Bob Wood.

Three people from Singular Publishing Group deserve special thanks: Sandy Doyle, Marie Linvill, and Sadanand Singh. They are always a pleasure to work with. Special thanks to Betty Lorich for typing the manuscript.

The senior author would like to acknowledge the felines who helped write this book: Chesia, Rapheal, Yoda, Ollie, Smokey, Homer, Myrtle, Rudi Jane, Lucky, Rudi II, Bobbi, and Sly. Tisha Pearl, Xela Sue, Bobby Joe, and Skeeter were equally helpful to the second author. Thanks are also due to Gina N. Easterly, Angela N. Tapp, Beth N. Witt, and Carol L. Yager for their contributions to this book.

CHAPTER 1

ETHICS AND ETHICAL VALUES

Adherence to ethical standards is essential to the assurance of high standards of professional practice. As the practices of speech-language pathology and audiology increase in complexity, the answers to ethical questions become equally complex and often debatable. Increased demands for accountability have prompted efforts to monitor and improve the quality of speech-language pathology and audiology services (Boston, 1994; Frattali, 1990–1991, 1991, 1992, 1994; Micheli, 1992; Theil, 1992).

Professional practice complaints and malpractice claims are investigated by speech-language pathologists, audiologists, attorneys, The American Speech-Language-Hearing Association (ASHA), the American Academy of Audiology (AAA), state associations, state licensure boards, and insurance companies. Study of such complaints and claims may identify potentially preventable sources of unprofessional conduct, unethical practice, and malpractice. Thus, knowledge about these complaints may alert speech-language pathologists and audiologists about practices that should be undertaken with caution.

Speech-language pathology and audiology tend to be low-risk professions. Unprofessional and/or unethical practice resulting in malpractice claims against speech-language pathologists and audiologists have been relatively low (ASHA, 1994f; Miller & Lubinski, 1986). The number of malpractice claims against speech-language pathologists and audiologists is relatively small in proportion to the number of practitioners (Suter & Coffman, 1986). However, being sued for malpractice is increasingly possible for the following reasons: (1) dramatic technological advances along with increased use of complex equipment and procedures; (2) involvement of more professionals and nonprofessionals in the total treatment of a client, thus increasing the risk of errors of communication and follow-up; (3) inadequate disciplinary action; (4) increase in the number of attorneys willing to take malpractice cases; (5) decreased tendency for consumers to treat professionals with the same reverence or respect as in the past; (6) increased entrepreneurial activity provides more opportunities to make money, increasing suspicion in the public eye; and (7) increases in the amount of damages awarded by jurors.

It is important that all professionals be aware of professional practice issues and develop skills in prevention and management of problems when they occur. The purposes of this chapter are (1) to identify ethical values, (2) to discuss ethical methods for dealing with situations encountered by students and practicing professionals in speech-language pathology and audiology, and (3) to identify external procedures for enforcing ethical practice.

ETHICS EDUCATION

Ethics were early established as a critical element in what eventually became the professions of speech-language pathology and audiology. When ASHA was founded as the American Academy of Speech Correction in 1925, the establishment of codes of ethics was identified as a primary reason for the organization. The maintaining of professional integrity was required of members by the first constitution of the organization.

When the constitution was revised in 1930, a major section was added that advised members of their responsibilities to the profession and to its members, of their obligation to keep patient information confidential, and to share information about methods and techniques. The revised constitution also included nine specific practices considered to be unethical. In 1948 a standing Committee on Ethical Practice was established (Paden, 1970). Appendix A provides a history of ASHA's ethics program spanning from 1925 through 1995.

Given ASHA's rich history of keeping ethics as a high priority, along with increased demands for accountability and quality management, there is growing agreement that professional ethics should be included in the education of speech-language pathologists and audiologists (Pannbacker, Lass, & Middleton, 1993; Pannbacker, Middleton, & Lass, 1994). Understanding and adhering to the standards for ethical practice is critical to the maintenance of professional autonomy for speech-language pathologists and audiologists. Thus, early exposure of speech-language pathology students to professional standards and ethics is important in their preparation as professionals (Green, 1986).

In recent years, ASHA committees have devoted time and effort to the formalized study of ethics.

1. ASHA has developed a manual of resource materials titled *Ethics: Resources for professional preparation and practice* (ASHA, 1994c).
2. ASHA's (1992a) long-range strategies plan for 1994 to 1999 includes expanding ". . . ethics education programs to professionals, clients, and ASHA employees" (p. 34).
3. ASHA's (1990b) standards for accreditation of education programs state ". . . the program must include instruction in the current ASHA Code of Ethics" (p. 94).
4. ASHA has sponsored an Ethics Colloquium and published the presentations as "Reflections on Ethics" (ASHA, 1990a).
5. ASHA's (1985) Committee on Supervision identified "Modeling and facilitating in . . . (the) ability to demonstrate ethical and legal conduct" as one of the 13 major tasks of supervision (p. 59).
6. ASHA has published two monographs that address issues in ethics (ASHA, 1992b, 1994d).

Although Asha has had an official Code of Ethics since 1930 and members have dealt with ethical dilemmas since that time, few speech-language pathologists and audiologists are required to take course work in ethics during their academic and clinical training. However, programs are addressing ethics in their curricula.

As AAA was not established until 1988, its ethics program has a shorter history. The Code of Ethics was first published in 1991 (AAA, 1991). Appendix B provides a history of AAA's ethics program spanning 1991 through 1995. The Code of Ethics republished in the Membership Directory in 1994 is unchanged (AAA, 1994–1995).

In a survey about ethics education in speech-language pathology, Pannbacker et al. (1993) found that discussions and lectures about ethics are the most frequently used methods of addressing ethics in academic and clinical training. Although over half, almost 57%, of the 144 program representatives responding to the survey felt course work on ethics should be required, only 13 of the programs surveyed offer an ethics course. Furthermore, the ethics course is required in only 6 of the programs, with the remaining 7 offering the course as an elective. A large majority of the programs surveyed, almost 85%, spend 20 hours or less in ethics training. The most important issues in ethics education identified in the survey were related to confidentiality, management decisions, professional competence, scope of practice, and practice standards.

Issues recently described in an ASHA (1992b) supplement on ethics and in ASHA's (1994c) ethics resources manual include: clinical practice by certificate holders in the profession in which they are not certified, competition, supervision of student clinicians, drawing cases for private practice from primary place of employment, fees for clinical services provided by students, and various issues about research and professional practice.

There are many ethical issues that warrant consideration. Programs in speech-language pathology and audiology are increasingly challenged to crowd more information into an already full curriculum. Modeling, role playing, or discussing various case situations or scenarios have been recommended as effective strategies for teaching ethics. Gonzalez and Coleman (1994) describe a student-led case study approach involving application of the Code of Ethics to relevant case scenarios.

Innovative ways of studying health care ethics have been used in medical education. Seedhouse (1991) described the use of simulations performed by drama students followed by practice with methodological ethical analysis, along with law lectures and small group discussions and case conferences. Case-based and issue-oriented ethics teaching were identified as the processes most used in Canadian medical schools (Baylis & Downie, 1991).

Bebeau, Rest, and Yamoor (1985) described the use of audio dramas in dental schools. Simulated teaching modules and techniques have been successfully integrated throughout the 2-year curriculum in an occupational therapy program (DeMars, Fleming, & Benham, 1991). Ryden, Duckett, Crisham, Caplan, and Schmitz (1989) and Mustapha and Seybert (1989) further emphasize the importance of integrating ethics into content throughout a nursing curriculum.

Other programs have elected to provide an intensive course on ethics. A two-credit course on biomedical ethics was credited as successfully improving moral reasoning of junior level allied health students as measured by Rest's Defining Issues Test (Glazer-Waldman, Hedl, & Chan, 1990).

The nursing profession has identified ethics as a topic warranting postgraduate continuing education among practicing nurses. O'Neil (1991) described a curriculum for a staff development program that includes mock case study presentations followed by review by a mock ethics committee.

The activities described require instructor time and commitment for planning and implementation. Spontaneous participatory activities are often unpredictable and are sometimes unclear and without complete closure. Such activities challenge the instructor who feels more comfortable dealing with factual information in a structured lecture style. In other words, teaching ethics is not easy. Computer simulation programs based on case situations have also been suggested as resourceful means of teaching ethics within an already crowded curriculum.

Ethics education, difficult as it may be, is justified (White, Hickson, Theriot, & Zaner, 1991). Lewis A. Barness, M.D., editor of *Advances in Pediatrics*, states that "Ethics is very personal, starting in the home" (Ledbetter, 1991, p. 365). However, the formal teaching of ethics to medical students, including the vocabulary of ethics, is well defended. Ledbetter (1991) concludes that "Medicine is best prioritized as a professional and ethical enterprise for the benefit of individuals and society, not a business to avoid conflicts of interest and self-serving practices" (p. 385).

Speech-language pathologists and audiologists need practical training in making ethical decisions that comply with the Codes of Ethics. Optimal training probably involves interactive discussions of situations that illustrate the principles of ASHA's and AAA's Codes of Ethics and some of the problems encountered when applying them to controversial issues. This book provides a series of scenarios or dilemmas for such discussions. Before considering the scenarios, however, it is important to define ethical values. Table 1–1 provides definitions of ethical values.

TABLE 1–1. Definition of Ethical Values

Term	Definition
Autonomy	A commitment to respect an individual's independent actions and choices.
Beneficence	An obligation to convey benefits and to help others to further their legitimate interests.
Confidentiality	An implicit understanding that information divulged by the patient to a professional will not be revealed to another person.
Harm avoidance (Nonmaleficence)	An obligation not to inflict evil, harm, or risk of harm on others.
Justice	An equal distribution of benefits and burdens and fair allocation of scarce resources.
Professional Responsibility	An obligation to observe the rules of professional conduct with patients, colleagues and the community at large.
Truth	The disclosure of all pertinent information including that which may reflect poorly on the informer.

Source: From "Assessment of Ethical Decisions and Values" by A. G. Rezler, R. L. Schwartz, S. S. Obenshain, P. Lambert, J. M. Gibson, and D. A. Bennahum, 1992, *Medical Education, 26,* 7–16.

ETHICAL VALUES

Autonomy is a commitment to respect an individual's independent actions and choices. AAA's Code of Ethics states that members shall respect the dignity, worth, and rights of those served. For example, possibly the most important members of a craniofacial team are the parents and patient, as they ultimately decide whether or not to follow the team's recommendations for management. Professionals must respect patients' choices. Sometimes it is not so clear-cut. Lesperance (1994) addresses the issue of the terminally ill patient's independent choice to die. Does that choice extend to the option of physician-assisted suicide? This is an issue of passionate debate. A review of medical oaths reveals that few manifest respect for patients' autonomy. Nonmalefi-cence, beneficence, justice, and confidentiality are most frequently included in the oaths (Dickstein, Erlen, & Erlen, 1991).

Rehabilitation teams sometimes struggle with a perceived incompatibility between client autonomy and beneficence. Altering the client's choice of outcomes or treatment objectives because the team concludes that the decision is in the best interests of the client is paternalistic (Purtilo, 1988). However, limited paternalism based on a rehabilitation team's careful, thoughtful deliberation about the best treatment(s) for a client to ultimately assure the heightening of client welfare may be justified (Purtilo, 1988). After all, rehabilitation means "making able again" and the process of rehabilitation includes restoring "functional abilities . . . [and] reaffirming, through rehabilitation, what makes this person a unique member of society" (Meier, 1988, p. 11).

Beneficence is an obligation to convey benefits and to help others further their legitimate interests. Certainly all professionals like to believe they are doing good for others when recommending and providing speech-language and audiology services. However, the benefits of such services must be appropriate, needed, and beneficial to the client and family. ASHA's Code of Ethics mandates that professionals hold paramount the welfare of the persons they serve professionally. AAA's Code of Ethics states that professionals shall exercise all reasonable precautions to avoid injury to persons in the delivery of services. Following is a discussion of factors that involve the welfare of clients and students served by speech-language pathologists and audiologists and examples of violations identified and published by ASHA's Ethical Practice Board (EPB) from 1985 through April, 1995 (see Tables 1–2 and 1–3).

The provision or supervision of clinical services without holding the appropriate certification was identified by the EPB in 38 instances. Most common in this group are those with certification in speech-language pathology (SLP) practicing audiology or those with certification in audiology (A) practicing speech-language pathology. Three of these individuals resorted to forgery.

One individual misrepresented preparation for dual certification and forged the program director's signature on the initial application for the cer-

TABLE 1–2. Number of Sanctions by Ethical Practice Violation and Year in *Asha* From 1985 Through April 1995

Ethical Practice Violation	1985	1986	1987	1988	1989	1990	1991	1992	1993	1994	1995	Total
Provided or supervised without appropriate certification or misrepresented credentials	10	11	2	5	3	0	1	0	3	3	0	38
Fraudulent Medicaid claim; charged for services not rendered; mail fraud	0	1	0	0	1	0	2	1	3	1	1	10
Incompetency; inaccurate or inadequate records; inadequate supervision of support personnel; improper clinical conduct/judgment; false claims, misleading statements	0	1	0	0	1	0	1	0	1	2	1	7
Rape, indecent exposure; assault conviction	0	0	0	1	0	0	1	0	2	0	0	4
Possession of stolen property	0	0	0	1	0	0	0	0	0	0	0	1
Photocopied National Exam	1	0	0	0	0	0	0	0	0	0	0	1
Total by Year	11	13	2	7	5	0	5	1	9	6	2	61

TABLE 1–3. Most Common Ethical Practice Violations in *Asha*. From 1985 Through April 1995

Principle of Ethics I, Rule A*	
Violation	Individuals should provide all services competently. Provided or supervised clinical services without holding the appropriate certificate.
Number of Violations	38
Principle of Ethics I, Rule A	Individuals shall provide all services competently.
Principle of Ethics I, Rule H	Individuals shall maintain adequate records of professional services rendered and products dispensed and shall allow access to these records when appropriately authorized.
Principle of Ethics I, Rule J	Individuals shall not charge for services not rendered nor shall they misrepresent, in any fashion, services rendered or products dispensed.
Principle of Ethics III, Rule C	Individuals shall not misrepresent diagnostic information, services rendered, or products dispensed or engage in any scheme or artifice to defraud in connection with obtaining payment or reimbursement for such services or products.
Violation	Charged for services not rendered, filed fraudulent Medicaid claims, made false claims/promises, made misleading statements, misrepresented results of clinical method, kept inadequate records.
Number of Violations	17
Principle of Ethics I	Individuals shall honor their responsibility to hold paramount the welfare of persons they serve professionally.
Violation	Convicted of rape, indecent exposure, indecent assault on a child.
Number of Violations	4
Principle of Ethics II, Rule D	The provision of support services may be delegated to persons who are neither certified nor in the certification process only when a certificate holder provides appropriate supervision.
Violation	Inadequately supervising support personnel.
Number of Violations	2

*Principles based on Code of Ethics Revised January 1, 1994.

tificates of clinical competence (CCC) (ASHA, 1989b). Another forged a CCC and an ASHA membership card, and a third forged a membership card by duplicating and altering the membership card of her Clinical Fellowship (CF) supervisor (ASHA, 1991a; 1994a)! What horrible false starts for those individuals' professional careers.

Failure to individualize programs or maintain high standards of competence and improperly delegating supportive personnel to services requiring a certified professional and/or making false claims or misleading statements were identified in seven instances. Such practices as citing false clinical information as fact, failing to administer appropriate tests or individualize instruction, and keeping inadequate records were all cited. The publication of false or exaggerated claims or promises and misleading statements about the results of clinical methods or benefits of products were identified in two of these instances. One individual promised a cure in his literature (ASHA, 1989a). Another was found guilty of fitting hearing aids over the phone (ASHA, 1994a). Clients should be able to decide about beginning therapy based on accurate information about the diagnosis, prognosis for improvement, and probable results of the recommended program or programs (Silverman, 1983).

When a subpoena is issued by a court for clinical records, professionals may find on careful review of those records such things as oversights, omissions, and regrettable statements. Having to supply records by subpoena tends to "sharpen one's meticulosity in keeping clinical records" (Flower, 1984, p. 280). Flower (1984) provides critical factors to consider when giving a deposition and when serving as a witness in a court proceeding.

Medical fraud or abuse is a concern to speech-language pathologists or audiologists. Reported problem areas in school settings include the speech-language pathologist and audiologist: (1) signing Medicaid claim forms for children they do not know and for whom they have never provided services; (2) signing Medicaid claim forms for children receiving services from persons who are not qualified providers and who are not being supervised by qualified providers; (3) providing services only to Medicaid-eligible children in the same school where non-Medicaid-eligible children receive services from providers who are not qualified; and (4) providing services to Medicaid-eligible children on an individual basis and providing only group services to non-Medicaid-eligible children, or providing Medicaid children with more frequent sessions (ASHA, 1994e).

Filing false Medicaid claims and charging for services not rendered have been cited in at least 10 instances. The EPB recently found one person guilty of charging for services rendered after a patient's recorded time of death (ASHA, 1994a). Possibly faulty record keeping contributed to these incidents.

Professionals who do not participate in continuing education by attending conventions, seminars, or workshops and by reading current monographs and journals are in violation of professional ethics. Knowledge about the most effective methods and techniques contribute to effective treatment and, hence, holding paramount the welfare of clients (Silverman, 1983). In addition, client welfare is further protected by the regular practice of evaluating treatment outcomes in an effort to capitalize on effective methods and modify or discard ineffective ones; when effective or ineffective methods are identified, clinicians are obligated to report these findings (Silverman, 1983).

ASHA's Code of Ethics states that "individuals shall not discriminate in the delivery of professional services on the basis of race or ethnicity, gender, age, religion, national origin, sexual orientation, or disability" (ASHA, 1994b, p. 1). Similarly, AAA's Code of Ethics states that "individuals . . . shall not discriminate in the provision of services to individuals on the basis of sex, race, religion, national origin, sexual orientation, or general health" (AAA, 1994–1995, p. 165). However, the issue of ability to pay is not addressed. Except in an emergency, some health care professions may refuse to serve certain individuals, such as Medicare or Medicaid clients, because they do not have the staff to do the necessary paperwork nor the cash flow to wait long periods of time for payment (Silverman, 1983). This factor opens questions of discrimination based on funding source.

The decision to remain silent about an incompetent colleague may be at the expense of client welfare. Principle of Ethics IV of ASHA's Code of Ethics states that "Individuals shall honor their responsibilities to the professions and their relationships with colleagues, students, and members of allied professions. Individuals shall uphold the dignity and autonomy of the professions, maintain harmonious interprofessional and intraprofessional relationships, and accept the professions' self-imposed standards" (ASHA, 1994b, p. 2). The decision to file malpractice claims against another professional is a serious one and requires that the claim be based only on objective, accurate information. However, client welfare must not be sacrificed by one professional protecting another from investigation (Flower, 1984). There are numerous advantages of the team approach to rehabilitation. However, faithfulness to colleagues may create a climate in which protection of colleagues may outweigh the obligation to client welfare (Purtilo, 1988).

Finally, it is the responsibility of every professional to maintain good mental and physical health, which implies being drug- and alcohol-free. The ASHA Code of Ethics, Principle I, Rule L states that "individuals whose professional services are adversely affected by substance abuse or other health related conditions shall seek professional assistance and, where appropriate, withdraw from the affected areas of practice" (ASHA, 1994b, p. 1).

Confidentiality is an implicit understanding that information divulged by the client to a professional will not be revealed to another person either orally or in writing. Unless required by law to do so, both ASHA's and AAA's Codes of Ethics mandate that individuals not reveal without authorization, any information about persons served professionally. ASHA's Code of Ethics adds the clause, "unless doing so is necessary to protect the welfare of the person or of the community" (ASHA, 1994b, p. 1).

There have been cases in which educators or health professionals have revealed information about possible child abuse only to have the claim disproved. This is a very difficult situation. When is the welfare of a client in question? The answer is not always clear. An example of breaching confidentiality to protect the community might involve informing authorities if a client reveals the intent to commit a crime (Silverman, 1983).

Harm avoidance, or nonmaleficence, is an obligation not to inflict evil, harm, or risk of harm on others. Silverman (1992) defines malpractice as "any type of negligent conduct by a professional that causes his or her patient (client) to be harmed either physically or emotionally" (p. 230). Malpractice includes: (1) misdiagnosis, (2) failure to reveal alternative treatment, (3) improper or substandard treatment, (4) failure to refer when appropriate, (5) referral to an inferior system for treatment, (6) breach of an active contract for service or for a product, (7) breach of an implied contract, (8) release of information to unauthorized persons, (9) failure to properly instruct in use of a potentially hazardous product, and (10) failure to warn of a potential hazard or harm (Rowland, 1988). Lynch (1986) described a number of risks from assessment or treatment, errors of omission, and misdiagnosis as well as actual harm and harm from unqualified practitioners.

Certainly the Ethical Practice Board is dealing with conduct that inflicts harm according to EPB reports about sexual misconduct with individuals served professionally. ASHA members have been sanctioned by the EPB because they were convicted of rape and/or indecent exposure or assault on a client (ASHA 1991c; 1993).

Full disclosure about research projects must be provided and permission given in an effort to avoid harm or discomfort to subjects. This is in compliance with Principle of Ethics I, Rule K that states, "Individuals shall use persons in research or as subjects of teaching demonstrations only with their informed consent" (ASHA, 1994b, p. 1). AAA's Code of Ethics requires full disclosure about the nature and possible effects of research or teaching activities to afford all persons informed free choice. An exception may be when the research involves the analysis of usual evaluation and therapy procedures that would have been carried out anyway as a part of the client's treatment (Flower, 1984).

Justice is an equal distribution of benefits and burdens and the fair allocation of scarce resources. With continued discussion about health care reform, it is important that focus be on inclusion of speech-language pathology and audiology services. It is also important that health care practices be based on what would best benefit the majority of Americans. AAA's Code of Ethics requires that "individuals shall not limit the delivery of professional services on any basis that is unjustifiable, or irrelevant to the need for the potential benefit from such services" (AAA, 1994–1995, p. 165). Speech-language pathologists and audiologists must be willing to make decisions to fund programs and/or projects that may not be directly related to their programs but that are needed for the good of the agency as a whole. One department, however, must not thrive at the expense of another. Also, it's important that in the spirit of team work, professionals be willing to help those who are carrying heavy workloads.

Professional responsibility is an obligation to observe the rules of professional conduct with clients, colleagues, and the community at-large. Certainly the Code of Ethics covers this area with the statement that "Individuals shall honor their responsibilities to the professions and their relationships with colleagues, students, and members of allied professions. Individuals shall uphold the dignity and autonomy of the professions, maintain harmonious interprofessional and intraprofessional relationships, and accept the professions' self-imposed standards" (ASHA, 1994b, p. 2). AAA's Code of Ethics includes similar statements.

Truth is the disclosure of all pertinent information, including those that may reflect poorly on the informer. The clinician might make an error that significantly impacts diagnostic findings or the results of clinical management. Certainly speech-language pathologists and audiologists are human and not infallible. In the interest of keeping consumers fully informed about the nature and possible effects of services, full disclosure is mandatory.

Both AAA and ASHA's Codes require accuracy in public statements about services and products as well as in representation of professional credentials. Further, both codes allow a reasonable prognostic statement but forbid a guarantee of results.

METHODS FOR DECISION MAKING

Dealing with ethical dilemmas requires careful study of basic ethical values followed by application to actual situations. Seymour (1994) advises the professional facing an ethical dilemma to first consult the Asha Code of Ethics (1994b) and Issues in Ethics Statements (ASHA, 1992b, 1994d). The AAA Code of Ethics (1994–1995) is an additional referral source for audiologists. If the answer remains unclear, Seymour further suggests that the professional seek advice from a supervisor, lawyer, state licensing board, or the Division of Ethics in the Asha National Office. Audiologists may also consult with the Ethical Practice Board of AAA. This is excellent advice.

In practice, Seymour and her students at the University of Massachusetts have developed a case study approach to increase student awareness about ethics and to provide students with practice in the ethical decision-making process. For guidance they use the Ethics Calibration Quick Test as they discuss various scenarios and attempt to resolve each dilemma. The Ethics Calibration Quick Test is an excellent tool for maintaining organized structure and focus in the deliberation process. An adaptation of Seymour's (1994) format is provided in Figure 1–1. As the scenarios in Chapter 2 are discussed, it

What is the problem/conflict/dilemma?

_____Is it a professional violation?
_____Is it a legal violation?
_____Is it both?

What values are in conflict?

_____Under the circumstances, what is of most value?
_____Will feelings interfere with judgment?

What evidence is available for objective consideration?

_____What parties are involved?
_____Have all parties been heard and all evidence considered?
_____Whose evidence is most convincing/believable?
_____Is there consistency in the evidence?
_____Has all available evidence been considered?
_____What is acceptable practice in this situation?

What action(s) can be taken or recommended?

_____Would outside consultation be beneficial?
If yes, from what source?
_____Define social, cultural, or political impact(s)
consequent to potential action(s).
_____Identify long and short term impact(s)
consequent to potential action(s).
_____Test each potential action for fairness.
_____Will the decision be fair to all involved?
(If yes, why? If not, why not?)

How will the decision impact the present and future?

_____How will the decision affect morale of parties involved?
_____How will the decision change how I feel about
myself as a person and as a professional?
_____How will the decision improve or deteriorate
present and future operations?

FIGURE 1–1. Identification and resolution of ethical dilemmas. (From "Ethical Considerations" by C. M. Seymour. In R. Lubinski and C. Frattali [Eds.], 1994, *Professional Issues in Speech-Language Pathology and Audiology* [pp. 61–64]. San Diego: Singular Publishing Group. Copyright 1994 by Singular Publishing Group. Reprinted with permission.)

is recommended that the dialogue follow this format in an effort to keep the discussion focused and to consider all aspects of the dilemma.

ETHICS ENFORCEMENT

The most effective means of enforcing ethical practice is by internal means or the voluntary commitment to ethical practice by every member of a profession. Fortunately the large majority of professions make every effort to engage in ethical and responsible clinical practice. To enforce ethical practice among those whose greed, ambition, or negligence evoke unethical practice, an external means of enforcement is necessary.

ASHA's Ethical Practice Board (EPB)

According to ASHA's Bylaws, the EPB has "the responsibility to interpret, administer, and enforce the Code of Ethics of the Association" (ASHA, 1994g, p. 3). The requirement that all ASHA members and those holding the certificates of clinical competence must fully comply with the Code of Ethics is the EPB's fundamental guiding principle.

EPB Procedures

It is the practice of the EPB to evaluate the merits of each case and to interpret the Code of Ethics as it applies to the individual incident. The procedures used by the board involve investigating the reported violation, generating and sending written notices and answers, imposing sanctions, providing disclosure to the membership, and reviewing the findings. Figure 1–2 provides an illustration of the procedures followed by the Ethical Practice Board.

Investigative procedures include careful review of each alleged violation of the Code of Ethics. For those cases the board decides to investigate, a letter is sent to the respondent outlining the allegation(s) and requiring a written response within 45 days. On review of the respondent's response, the EPB may determine insufficient evidence to support the allegation(s) and advise the respondent and the complainant of this decision. If the EPB finds sufficient evidence to proceed, then the specific violation of the Code of Ethics is determined and the respondent is notified to cease and desist from the practice. If the respondent does not comply, then sanctions are invoked.

All written notices and answers are sent certified mail to the addressee with a request for return receipt. The respondent is provided with the initial findings by the board and given the opportunity to request within 30 days fur-

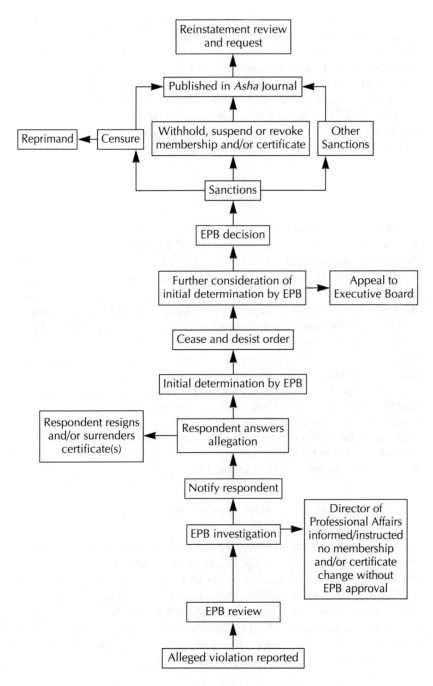

FIGURE 1–2. ASHA's Ethical Practice Board procedure.

ther consideration by the EPB. The respondent may provide additional written documentation or may appear personally with counsel or by a conference telephone call to present evidence at an informal hearing of the EPB for further consideration of the case. On notification of the decision by the EPB following a hearing for further consideration, the respondent may appeal the decision within 30 days to ASHA's Executive Board, providing that the decision made by the EPB required revocation of membership and/or certification or disclosure of the sanction in the *Asha* journal. The appeal must specify how and why the EPB decision was allegedly wrong.

Sanctions

Possible sanctions include reprimand; censure; withhold, suspend, or revoke membership; withhold, suspend, or revoke the certificate(s); or any other sanctions deemed appropriate by the EPB. Since February 1985, the names of individuals found in violation of the Code of Ethics, when the sanction is censure or revocation of membership or certification, are disclosed to the membership and public in the *Asha* journal. The number of published sanctions is small but has fluctuated widely from a low of none in 1990 to a high of 13 in 1986. The average number of sanctions per year is five. The most frequent sanction was revocation of membership, and the second most frequent was revocation of both membership and certification (see Table 1–4).

After 1 year and a two-thirds vote of the EPB, an individual's membership or certification may be reinstated, if there is adequate evidence that the cause of the sanction(s) has been rectified and that the individual will abide by the Code of Ethics in the future. The EPB must make this decision based on the "premise that reinstatement is in the best interest of the Association and of persons served professionally" (ASHA, 1994g, p. 5).

State Associations

Forty-nine of the 50 states (excluding Alaska) have state speech-language-hearing associations (SSHA). For the SSHA to be recognized by ASHA it must submit required information to ASHA every 5 years. The purposes of the SSHA and the SSHA's membership requirements must be consistent with ASHA's purposes and requirements (ASHA, 1991b). One of the requirements is a Code of Ethics for the SSHA. Therefore, ethics enforcement may also occur as a function of the SSHA. Procedures vary among states, but should be similar to the procedures described for ASHA's Ethical Practice Board.

TABLE 1–4. Actions of the Ethical Practice Board Published in Asha

Year (Month)	Asha Vol/Pg	Number Actions	Gender M	Gender F	Withhold/Revoke Membership/ Certification	Censure	Reprimand
1985 (February)	27 49	5	0	5	5	0	0
1985 (May)	27 45	4	3	1	3	1	0
1985 (September)	27 65	1	0	1	1	0	0
1985 (December)	27 55	1	0	1	1	0	0
1986 (February)	28 45	5	2	3	4	0	1
1986 (June)	28 69	1	0	1	1	0	0
1986 (July)	28 51	4	2	2	4	0	0
1986 (November)	28 58	3	2	1	2	1	0
1987 (April)	29 62	2	1	1	2	0	0
1988 (January)	30 59	4	1	3	4	0	0
1988 (September)	30 79	3	1	2	3	0	0
1989 (September)	31 47	2	1	1	2	0	0
1989 (November)	31 59	3	0	3	2	1	0
1991 (January)	33 68	2	1	1	1	1	0
1991 (April)	33 70	1	0	1	1	0	0
1991 (August)	33 55	1	1	0	1	0	0

(continued)

TABLE 1–4. *(continued)*

Year (Month)	Asha Vol/Pg	Number Actions	Gender M	F	Withhold/Revoke Membership/Certification	Censure	Reprimand
1991 (December)	33 12	1	1	0	1	0	0
1992 (August)	34 17	1	0	1	1	0	0
1993 (January)	35 12	1	1	0	0	1	0
1993 (April)	35 23	5	4	1	3	2	0
1993 (August)	35 16	3	0	3	1	2	0
1994 (February)	36 15	2	0	2	1	1	0
1994 (May)	36 16	1	0	1	1	0	0
1994 (August)	36 22	3	2	1	2	1	0
1995 (April)	37 33	2	2	2	0	2	1
Totals		61	23	38	47	13	1
			38%	62%	77%	21%	2%

AAA's Ethical Practice Board

A complaint received by AAA's Ethical Practice Board should be reported in letter format with documentation sufficient to support the alleged violation. AAA's EPB requests that complainants sign a Waiver of Confidentiality so that the name of the complainant can be revealed if it is necessary during the investigation. After the complaint is thoroughly investigated, it is reviewed by the members of the EPB and a finding is reached regarding infractions of the code. AAA members found in violation of the code may appeal the decision of the EPB to the Executive Committee of the academy.

Sanctions

Possible sanctions include: reprimand, cease and desist order, suspension of membership, and revocation of membership. Notification of a reprimand is limited to the member and the complainant. A cease and desist order may be published on a two-thirds vote of the Ethical Practice Board. Both the suspension of membership and the revocation of membership are reported in the official publications of the academy.

AAA's Ethical Practice Board has received several complaints about the use of degrees before the public or peers from nonaccredited universities or in nonrelated fields (T. N. Decker, personal communication, May 18, 1995). Complaints have been received concerning advertising as well. These complaints have been handled confidentially without published sanctions in AAA's journals. However, the EPB has requested that the Executive Board publish an "Issues in Ethics" article on this issue in a future journal. An additional "Issues in Ethics" article will be published on conflict of interest, which will parallel ASHA's article on the topic (ASHA, 1994d).

State Licensure Boards

State licensure laws have prohibitions against unprofessional conduct, including misrepresentation, negligence, and other infringements. Complaints about unprofessional conduct are made to state licensing boards. These boards have the power to suspend or revoke a license to practice speech-language pathology or audiology in that state (Koop, 1994). In a study of state licensing boards, Miller and Lubinski (1986) found the most frequent complaints were: practicing without a license, practicing beyond the scope permitted by law, and incorrect or inadequate treatment. Graff (1992) indicated the most frequent complaints were about advertising, fraud, and unprofessional conduct. Other complaints included inappropriate standard of care, unethical practice, refusal of service, and inadequate record keeping.

Occupational licensing is an exercise of the state's power to protect the health, safety and welfare of its citizens. Forty-three states have licensure laws that govern the practices of audiologists and/or speech-language pathologists. In a variety of ways within these laws, ethical practice is given the force of law. Some states, like Utah, make a simple statement that it is a requirement for licensure to "be in compliance with the regulations of conduct and codes of ethics for the profession of speech-language pathology and audiology" (SLP and Aud Licensing Act, 1994, p. 4). Other states like Kentucky, Louisiana, Oregon, and North Carolina, which pattern their Codes of Ethics on ASHA's, have more complex codes (Kentucky Board of Speech-Language Pathology and Audiology, 1994; Louisiana Board of Examiners for Speech Pathology and Audiology, 1991; Oregon, 1994; Licensure Act-NC, 1989). One problem with this is that ASHA revises and updates the Code of Ethics frequently. State law is not so easily revised. For example, North Carolina's Code of Ethics is based on a version of ASHA's that held the "bundling" of fees for products dispensed and services rendered as unethical. This is no longer considered unethical behavior, but could lead to sanctioning in a state with rules patterned on this older version of ASHA's Code of Ethics.

Kentucky, Louisiana, and Oregon also pattern their Codes of Ethics on a version that predates the current one. These codes are more confusing to follow, as they are divided into principles of ethics, ethical proscriptions, and matters of professional propriety. ASHA's current code more simply describes principles of ethics that form an underlying moral basis, followed by rules of ethics that are statements of minimally acceptable professional conduct.

Regulations for ethical behaviors are found in various locations within individual state laws. Sometimes these regulations are found in the body of the law, in the Administrative Code, in the Rules, or in the Rules and Regulations.

Practicing speech-language pathologists and audiologists who work in states that require licensure should have and refer to a current copy of the State's law and the rules and regulations. Familiarity with and adherence to the ethical practice requirements of the law are important to maintaining a license to practice one's profession.

Sanctions

Almost all states have the power to suspend or revoke a license for an ethical violation. A few have the authority to levy a fine. Many states can place a licensee on probation, issue a public or private reprimand, issue cease and desist orders, and refuse to issue or renew a license.

SUMMARY

The framing of a professional code of ethics was a high priority activity assigned to members of the American Speech and Hearing Association in

1925 and more recently of the American Academy of Audiology established in 1988. Asha's code has evolved over the years to reflect changes in accepted practices within the professions of speech-language pathology and audiology. The expanding complexity of these professions has been accompanied by increasingly debatable ethical practice questions. Thus, growing attention is given to ethics education in the university setting and to continuing education about ethics for practicing professionals.

Included in ethics education is a study of ethical values. Published violations of code(s) of ethical practice reveal the need for a better understanding of the ethical values underlying professional codes of ethical practice. Potentially brilliant careers of fully credentialed professionals can be severely damaged by poor judgment involving questions of ethical practice.

The Ethical Practice Boards of the American Speech-Language-Hearing Association and the American Academy of Audiology review reported ethical violations and may impose various sanctions. State associations and state licensure boards also have programs for enforcing their codes of ethical practice.

The image of a profession and of individual professionals involves voluntary commitment to ethical practice by every member. Ethical decision making requires careful study of ethical values followed by application of those values to actual situations. Such decision making should follow a structured format so that all aspects of any dilemma in question are considered. Ethics education provides the tools for an ethical outcome to ethical quandaries professionals increasingly face.

REFERENCES

American Academy of Audiology. (1991). Code of Ethics. *Audiology Today,* *3*(1), 14–16.

American Academy of Audiology. (1994–1995). Code of ethics. *American Academy of Audiology Membership Directory*, 165–169.

American Speech-Language-Hearing Association. (1985, June). Clinical supervision in speech-language pathology and audiology. *Asha, 27*, 57–60.

American Speech-Language-Hearing Association. (1989a, September). Actions of the Ethical Practice Board. *Asha, 31*, 47.

American Speech-Language-Hearing Association. (1989b, November). Actions of the Ethical Practice Board. *Asha, 31*, 59.

American Speech-Language-Hearing Association. (1990a). *Reflections on ethics.* Rockville, MD: Author.

American Speech-Language-Hearing Association. (1990b, June). Standards for accreditation of educational programs. *Asha, 32*, 93–94, 100.

American Speech-Language-Hearing Association. (1991a, April). Actions of the Ethical Practice Board. *Asha, 33*, 70.

American Speech-Language-Hearing Association. (1991b). Bylaws and 1988 deletion from bylaws of the American Speech-Language-Hearing Association, Rockville, MD: Author.

American Speech-Language-Hearing Association. (1991c, January). Ethical Practice Board Actions, *Asha, 33*, 68.

American Speech-Language-Hearing Association. (1992a, May). Asha's proposed long range strategic plan. *Asha, 34*, 32–36.

American Speech-Language-Hearing Association. (1992b). Issues in ethics. *Asha, 34*(March, Suppl. 9), 3–21.

American Speech-Language-Hearing Association. (1993, April). Actions of the Ethical Practice Board. *Asha, 35*, 23.

American Speech-Language-Hearing Association. (1994a, August). Actions of the Ethical Practice Board. *Asha, 36*, 22.

American Speech-Language-Hearing Association. (1994b). Code of Ethics. *Asha, 36*(Suppl. 13), 1–2.

American Speech-Language-Hearing Association. (1994c). *Ethics: Resources for professional preparation and practice*. Rockville, MD: Author.

American Speech-Language-Hearing Association. (1994d). Issues in ethics. *Asha, 36*(Suppl. 13), 7–27.

American Speech-Language-Hearing Association. (1994e). Medicaid issues for public school practitioners. *Asha, 34*(8), 31–32.

American Speech-Language-Hearing Association. (1994f). Professional liability and risk management for audiology and speech-language pathology professions. *Asha, 36*(Suppl. 12), 25–38.

American Speech-Language-Hearing Association. (1994g). Statement of practices and procedures. *Asha, 36*(Suppl. 13), 3–5.

Baylis, F., & Downie, J. (1991). Ethics education for Canadian medical students. *Academic Medicine, 66*(7), 413–414.

Bebeau, M. J., Rest, J. R., & Yamoor, C. M. (1985). Measuring dental students' ethical sensitivity. *Journal of Dental Education, 49*(4), 225–235.

Boston, B. O. (1994). Destiny is in the data: A wake-up call for outcome measures. *Asha, 36*(11), 35–38.

DeMars, P. A., Fleming, J. D., & Benham, P. A. (1991). Ethics across the occupational therapy curriculum. *American Journal of Occupational Therapy, 45*(9), 782–787.

Dickstein, E., Erlen, J., & Erlen, J. A. (1991). Ethical principles contained in currently professed medical oaths. *Academic Medicine, 66*(10), 622–624.

Flower, R. M. (1984). *Delivery of speech-language pathology and audiology services*. Baltimore, MD: Williams and Wilkins.

Frattali, C. M. (1990–1991). In pursuit of quality: Evaluating clinical outcomes. *National Student Speech-Language-Hearing Association Journal, 18*(1), 4–16.

Frattali, C. M. (1991). From quality assurance to total quality management. *American Journal of Audiology, 1*, 41–47.

Frattali, C. M. (1992). Total quality management: Striving for continuous improvement. *Hearsay, 7*(1), 4–8, 21.

Frattali, C. M. (1994). Quality improvement. In R. Lubinski & C. M. Frattali (Eds.), *Professional issues in speech-language pathology and audiology* (pp. 246–259). San Diego: Singular Publishing Group.

Glazer-Waldman, H. R., Hedl, J. J., & Chan, F. (1990). Impacting moral reasoning in allied health students. *Journal of Allied Health, 19,* 351–360.

Gonzalez, L. S., & Coleman, R. O. (1994). Ethics education: Students prefer the case study approach. *Asha, 36*(8), 47–48.

Graff, L. L. (1992). Speech-language pathologists and audiologists: Professional liability. Poster session presented at the 1992 annual convention of the American Speech-Language Hearing Association, San Antonio, TX.

Green, W. W. (1986). Professional standards and ethics. In R. McLauchlin (Ed.), *Speech-language pathology and audiology* (pp. 135–158). NY: Grune & Stratton.

Kentucky Board of Speech-Language Pathology and Audiology. (1994). Commonwealth of Kentucky Laws and Regulations for Speech-Language Pathologists and Audiologists. Frankfort, KY: Author.

Koop, R. (1994). Professional liability. In R. Lubinski & C. M. Frattali (Eds.), *Professional issues in speech-language pathology and audiology* (pp. 166–172). San Diego: Singular Publishing Group.

Ledbetter, E. O. (1991). Ethics education in medicine. *Advances in Pediatrics, 38,* 365–386.

Lesperance, K. (1994, June 27). Ethics in Medicine: Do patients' rights extend to aid in dying? *ADVANCE for Speech-Language Pathologists & Audiologists,* 18–19.

Licensure Act for Speech and Language Pathologists and Audiologists. (1989). North Carolina Statutory Authority, §§150B-40; 90-304. (1977 and amended 1989).

Louisiana Board of Examiners for Speech Pathology and Audiology. (1991). Rules and Regulations. Baton Rouge: Bourque Printing, Inc.

Lynch, D. (1986). Harm to the public: Is it real? *Asha, 28*(6), 25–31.

Meier, R. H. (1988). Recent developments in rehabilitation giving rise to important new (and old) ethical issues and concerns. *American Journal of Physical Medicine & Rehabilitation, 67,* 7–11.

Micheli, S. (1992). The name of the game is . . . documentation. *Hearsay, 7*(1), 22–24.

Miller, T. D., & Lubinski, R. (1986). Professional liability in speech-language pathology and audiology. *Asha, 28*(6), 45–47.

Mustapha, S., & Seybert, J. (1989). Moral reasoning in college students: Implications for nursing education. *Journal of Nursing Education, 28*(3), 107–111.

O'Neil, J. A. (1991). Teaching basic ethical concepts and decision-making: A staff development application. *Journal of Continuing Education in Nursing, 22*(5), 184–188.

Oregon Administrative Rules, Board of Examiners for Speech Pathology and Audiology. (1994, August) Stat. ORS681.340, 681.420 & 681.460. (1990).

Paden, E. (1970). *A history of the American Speech and Hearing Association: 1925–1958.* Washington, DC: American Speech and Hearing Association.

Pannbacker, M., Lass, N. J., & Middleton, G. F. (1993, April). Ethics education in speech-language pathology training programs. *Asha, 35,* 53–55.

Pannbacker, M. H., Middleton, G. F., & Lass, N. J. (1994, September). Ethics education for speech-language pathologists and audiologists. *Asha, 36,* 40–43.

Purtilo, R. B. (1988). Ethical issues in teamwork: The context of rehabilitation. *Archives of Physical Medicine Rehabilitation, 69,* 318–322.

Rezler, A. G., Schwartz, R. L., Obenshain, S. S., Lambert, P., Gibson, J. M., & Bennahum, D. A. (1992). *Medical Education, 26,* 7–16.

Rowland, R. C. (1988). Malpractice in audiology and speech-language pathology. *Asha, 30*(1), 45–48.

Ryden, M. B., Duckett, L., Crisham, P., Caplan, A., & Schmitz, K. (1989). Multi-course sequential learning as a model for content integration: Ethics as a prototype. *Journal of Nursing Education, 28*(3), 102–106.

Seedhouse, D. F. (1991). Health care ethics teaching for medical students. *Medical Education, 25,* 230–237.

Seymour, C. M. (1994). Ethical considerations. In R. Lubinski & C. Frattali (Eds.), *Professional issues in speech-language pathology and audiology* (pp. 61–74). San Diego: Singular Publishing Group.

Silverman, F. H. (1983). *Legal aspects of speech-language pathology and audiology.* Englewood Cliffs, NJ: Prentice Hall.

Silverman, F. H. (1992). *Legal-ethical considerations, restrictions, and obligations for clinicians who treat communicative disorders.* Springfield, IL: Charles C. Thomas.

Speech-Language Pathology and Audiology Licensing Act. (1994, May). Utah Code Annotated 1953 as Amended by Session Laws of Utah 1994. §§58-41-1-16. (1953 and amended 1994).

Suter, A. H., & Coffman, S. V. (1986). Legal aspects. In R. M. McLauchlin (Ed.), *Speech-language pathology and audiology: Issues and management* (pp. 355–380). New York: Grune & Stratton.

Theil, C. M. (1992). Developing a comprehensive, manageable quality improvement program. *Hearsay, 7*(1), 28–33.

White, B. D., Hickson, G. B., Theriot, R., & Zaner, R. M. (1991). A medical ethics issues survey of residents in five pediatric training programs. *American Journal of Diseases of Children, 145,* 161–164.

C H A P T E R   2

ACADEMIC CASE STUDIES

This chapter describes ethical dilemmas from academia. The ASHA (1994) Code of Ethics Principle I states "Individuals shall honor their responsibility to hold paramount the welfare of persons they serve professionally" (p. 1). AAA's (1994–1995) Code of Ethics Principle 1 similarly states "members shall provide professional services with honesty and compassion, and shall respect the dignity, worth and rights of those served" (p. 165). For faculty and supervisors in speech-language pathology and audiology training programs, this includes students as well as clients. Case studies from academia are summarized in Table 2–1, and cover such topics as cheating, insufficient and/or unfair supervision, irresponsible mentoring, biased student ratings, noncom-

TABLE 2–1. Summary of Academic Case Studies

Page	Title and Topic	Concepts and Issue
27	Biased Student Ratings	Harmonious professional relationships
29	Biased Textbook Selection	Conflict of interest
30	Cheating 1 and Cheating 2	Academic honesty
33	Conflict of Interest	Doctoral student reviews advisor's book
35	Demonstration Without Consent	Video of client without permission

(continued)

TABLE 2–1. *(continued)*

Page	Title and Topic	Concepts and Issue
36	Discrimination	Sexual orientation
37	Disharmony Among Students	Relationship with colleagues
38	Faulty File Management	Failure to protect confidentiality and comply with accreditation standards
39	Grades Over Client Welfare	Welfare of client; responsibility in relationships with colleagues
40	Inappropriate Attire	Unprofessional appearance
41	Inappropriate Credential to Supervise	Audiologist supervises speech-language practicum
43	Independent Referral by Student	Failure to hold appropriate credential; outside scope of competence
44	Inflated Grading	Honest assignment of grade(s)
45	Information Exposure	Failure to keep information confidential
46	Insufficient Supervision	Inadequate supervision
47	Interprofessional Relationships	Inaccurate information
48	Irresponsible Mentor	Professional responsibility
49	Licensed Assistant	Lack of certification
50	Misrepresentation of Credentials	Inappropriate use of the title speech-language pathologist
51	No Available Supervisor	Certified supervisor not available
52	Off-Site Practicum Compliance	Allowing violation of Code of Ethics
54	Paid Clinical Practicum	Violation of clinical practicum experience and supervision standards
55	Plagiarizing a Diagnostic Report	Misconduct
56	Poor Professional Relationships	Negative comments about public schools
57	Salary Compression	Honesty about remuneration
59	Self-Referrals	Conflict of interest

TABLE 2–1. *(continued)*

Page	Title and Topic	Concepts and Issue
60	Self-Serving Authority	Conflict of interest
61	Student Clinician Complaints	Conduct that could adversely reflect on supervisor
62	Student in Private Practice	Failure to hold appropriate credential
63	Time Commitment Conflict	Conflict of interest; welfare of client
64	Treatment Efficacy vs. Student Training	Ineffective treatment
65	Uncertified Supervisor	Irresponsible professional conduct
67	Unfair and Insufficient Supervision	Inadequate supervision
68	Unfair Treatment of Supervisee	Confidentiality; prevailing professional standards
69	Unlicensed Faculty Practice Plan Member	Clinical practice without licensure; conflict of interest; state versus ASHA jurisdiction
70	Unprepared for Treatment	Failure to prepare for treatment; welfare of client

pliance of off-campus practicum with certification and accreditation requirements, and biased selection of textbooks.

BIASED STUDENT RATINGS

You are the instructor for a new course in audiology at a state university. At the end of the semester one of the students' written comments about the course is, "I feel that the program's faculty has a very poor attitude toward this class. The faculty members that I spoke with seem to feel that it is ridiculous that we are getting credit for the course and even more ridiculous that we are being graded."

Areas of ASHA's Code of Ethics That May Apply

Principle of Ethics IV, Rules A, B, and D

Areas of AAA's Code of Ethics That May Apply

Principle 5, Rule 5c
Principle 8, Rule 8b

Possible Solutions

1. Do nothing.
2. Discuss the student's comment and provide copies of the course syllabus at a faculty meeting.
3. Discuss the comment with the program director.

Discussion Questions

1. Is there a lack of cohesion between speech-language pathology and audiology faculty?
2. How can this be avoided in the future?
3. Does the course in question need revision?

Background Information

Broder, J. M., & Dorfman, J. H. (1994). Determinants of teaching quality: What's important to students? *Research in Higher Education, 35*(2), 235–249.

Goldman, L. (1993). On the erosion of education and the eroding foundations of teacher education (or why we should not take student evaluation of faculty seriously). *Teacher Education Quarterly, 20*(2), 57–64.

Goodwin, L. D., & Stevens, E. A. (1993). The influence of gender on university faculty members' perceptions of "good" teaching. *Journal of Higher Education, 64*(2), 166–185.

Hansen, W. L. (1993). Bringing total quality improvement into the college classroom. *Higher Education, 25*(3), 259–279.

Hativa, N., & Raviv, A. (1993). Using a single score for summative evaluation by students. *Research in Higher Education, 34*(5), 625–646.

Marsh, H. W., & Bailey, M. (1993). Multidimensional students' evaluations of teaching effectiveness. *Journal of Higher Education, 64*(1), 1–18.

Watkins, D. (1994). Student evaluations of university teaching: A cross-cultural perspective. *Research in Higher Education, 35*(2), 251–266.

BIASED TEXTBOOK SELECTION

A faculty member in audiology usually selects textbooks written by himself or his friends.

Areas of ASHA's Code of Ethics That May Apply

Principle of Ethics III, Rule C and E
Principle of Ethics IV, Rule D

Areas of AAA's Code of Ethics That May Apply

Principle 5, Rules 5a and 5c
Principle 6, Rule 6b
Principle 7, Rules 7a and 7b

Possible Solutions

1. Evaluate criteria for selecting textbooks.
2. Review student evaluations of course, including textbook selection.
3. Consider adoption of other textbooks.
4. Discuss appearance of impropriety with faculty member.
5. Faculty member donates royalties of books sold to local students to a university or program scholarship fund.

Discussion Questions

1. What criteria were used to select textbooks?
2. How can textbooks be evaluated?
3. Why should student input be obtained in selecting textbooks?
4. How does academic freedom impact textbook selection?

Background Information

Blancett, S. S. (1988). Approaches to evaluating textbooks and media. *Nurse Educator, 13*(1), 6–7.

Grosskopf, D. (1981). Textbook evaluation and selection in the curriculum. *Nurse Educator, 6*, 32–35.

McLeod, P. J. (1986). Faculty evaluation of medical textbooks and optional readings. *Journal of Medical Education, 61*, 608–609.

Phillips, C. G., & Harman, E. (1986). Criteria for selecting textbooks. *Nurse Educator, 11*(2), 31–34.

Sellers, S. C., & Haag, B. A. (1993). A nursing textbook evaluation instrument for multicultural, nonsexist concepts. *Educational Innovations, 32*(6), 270–272.

Wakefield-Fisher, M. (1986). How to evaluate nursing textbooks. *Nursing Outlook, 34*(2), 72–73, 98.

CHEATING—1

Students in the final clinical practicum before graduation were required to develop a scholarly paper on a current clinical issue. A student submitted a previously written paper on the topic. This paper was an exact copy of one previously submitted by the student for another course requirement.

Areas of ASHA's Code of Ethics That May Apply

Principle of Ethics IV, Rule B

Areas of AAA's Code of Ethics That May Apply

Principle 8, Rule 8b

Possible Solutions

1. Inform students of faculty expectations concerning course work and of school policies regarding academic dishonesty.
2. Give student a failing grade, which means that graduation requirements are not met.
3. Require that student repeat practicum, with a delay in graduation.
4. Review university/department Honor Code.

Discussion Questions

1. How was it determined that the papers were duplicates?
2. What was the student's explanation for this duplication?

3. How should the clinical faculty respond?

4. Are honor codes usually effective in controlling cheating? What are some of the factors that might reduce the effectiveness of an honor code?

Background Information

Anderson, M. (1992). *Impostors in the temple.* New York: Simon and Schuster.

Anderson, R. W., & Obenshain, S. S. (1994). Cheating by students: Findings, reflections, and remedies. *Academic Medicine, 69*(5), 323–331.

Booth, D. E., & Hoyer, P. J. (1992). Cheating: Faculty responsibilities when integrity fails. *Nursing Outlook, 40*(2), 86–93.

Bradshaw, M. J., & Lowenstein, A. J. (1990). Perspectives on academic dishonesty. *Nurse Educator, 15*(5), 10–15.

Falleur, D. (1990). An investigation of academic dishonesty in allied health: Incidence and definitions. *Journal Allied Health, 19*(3), 313–325.

McCabe, D. L., & Trevino, L. K. (1993). Academic dishonesty: Honor codes and other contextual influences. *Journal of Higher Education, 64*(5), 522–538.

Mowrer, D. E. (1994). Cooperative learning: New roles for students and professors. *National Student Speech-Language-Hearing Association Journal, 21*, 82–86.

Ozar, D. T. (1991). The ethical ramifications of cheating. *Journal of Dental Education, 55*(4), 276–281.

Rozanie, C. P. (1991). Cheating in medical schools: Implications for students and patients. *Journal of the American Medical Association, 266*(17), 2453–2456.

Simpson, D. E., Yindra, K. J., Towne, J. B., & Rosenfeld, P. S. (1989). Medical students' perceptions of cheating. *Academic Medicine, 64*(3), 221–222.

Stern, E. B., & Haulicek, L. (1986). Academic misconduct: Results of faculty and undergraduate surveys. *Journal of Allied Health, 15*(2), 129–142.

Wagner, R. F. (1993). Medical student academic misconduct: Implications of recent case law and possible institutional responses. *Academic Medicine, 68*(12), 887–889.

CHEATING—2

A student with poor class attendance asks to go to the restroom during an examination. You are in the restroom during the exam and notice the student consulting notes left there. You are a speech-language pathology major but are not now in the class that is taking the exam. What would you do?

Areas of ASHA's Code of Ethics That May Apply

Principle of Ethics II, Rule C
Principle of Ethics IV, Rules B and C

Areas of AAA's Code of Ethics That May Apply

Principle 2, Rule 2e
Principle 8, Rules 8b and 8c

Possible Solutions

1. Report the matter to the instructor who gave the examination.
2. Tell the student that the act is in violation of university policy on academic honesty.
3. Report the matter to the Dean of Students.
4. Look the other way.

Discussion Questions

1. Whose responsibility is it to prevent cheating?
2. Should the instructor have allowed the student to leave the room during the examination?
3. Is cheating a small or significant problem in universities?
4. Is there too much competition to achieve high grades?
5. How might cheating be reduced or avoided in the university setting?
6. Is cheating in speech-language pathology and audiology classes a violation of ASHA's Principle I and AAA's Principle 1, holding paramount the welfare of persons served professionally?

Background Information

Anderson, M. (1992). *Impostors in the temple*. New York: Simon and Schuster.

Anderson, R. W., & Obenshain, S. S. (1994). Cheating by students: Findings, reflections, and remedies. *Academic Medicine, 69*(5), 323–331.

Booth, D. E., & Hoyer, P. J. (1992). Cheating: Faculty responsibilities when integrity fails. *Nursing Outlook, 40*(2), 86–93.

Bradshaw, M. J., & Lowenstein, A. J. (1990). Perspectives on academic dishonesty. *Nurse Educator, 15*(5), 10–15.

Falleur, D. (1990). An investigation of academic dishonesty in allied health: Incidence and definitions. *Journal of Allied Health, 19*(3), 313–325.

McCabe, D. L., & Trevino, L. K. (1993). Academic dishonesty: Honor codes and other contextual influences. *Journal of Higher Education, 64*(5), 522–538.

Mowrer, D. E. (1994). Cooperative learning: New roles for students and professors. *National Student Speech-Language-Hearing Association Journal, 21*, 82–86.

Ozar, D. T. (1991). The ethical ramifications of cheating. *Journal of Dental Education, 55*(4), 276–281.

Rozanie, C. P. (1991). Cheating in medical schools: Implications for students and patients. *Journal of the American Medical Association, 266*(17), 2453–2456.

Simpson, D. E., Yindra, K. J., Towne, J. B., & Rosenfeld, P. S. (1989). Medical students' perceptions of cheating. Academic *Medicine, 64*(3), 221–222.

Stern, E. B., & Haulicek, L. (1986). Academic misconduct: Results of faculty and undergraduate surveys. *Journal Allied Health, 15*(2), 129–142.

Wagner, R. F. (1993). Medical student academic misconduct: Implications of recent case law and possible institutional responses. *Academic Medicine, 68*(12), 887–889.

CONFLICT OF INTEREST

An audiologist who is a doctoral candidate publishes a review in a professional journal of the candidate's academic advisor's recently published book. The review is not critical—that is, only strengths are identified and no weaknesses are recognized.

Areas of ASHA's Code of Ethics That May Apply

Principle of Ethics III, Rules B and E
Principle of Ethics IV, Rule D

Areas of AAA's Code of Ethics That May Apply

Principle 5, Rule 5a
Principle 6, Rule 6b
Principle 7, Rule 7b

Possible Solutions

1. Discuss the review with the doctoral candidate and express your concern.
2. Discuss the review with the doctoral candidate's academic advisor.
3. Write a letter to the editor of the journal in which the book review was published.
4. Do nothing and pretend it did not happen.
5. Generate critical and objective appraisal of the book in a second review by someone who is knowledgeable about the topic.

Discussion Questions

1. Could this be a conflict of interest? Would disclosure of the reviewer's affiliation with the work matter?
2. How could the doctoral student impartially review a book authored by the candidate's academic advisor?
3. Would it matter if the review had been solicited by the journal or was unsolicited?
4. Is this review in agreement with other reviews of the same book?
5. What would be the criteria for determining if the review is biased?
6. How can possible paternalism, personal opinion, and biases be avoided in reviews of the literature?
7. Which is of more concern in this situation, an apparent conflict of interest or the appearance of a conflict of interest?

Background Information

American Speech-Language-Hearing Association. (1994). Conflicts of professional interest. *Asha, 36*(Suppl. 13), 7–8.

American Speech-Language-Hearing Association. (1994). Ethics in research and professional practice. *Asha, 36*(Suppl. 13), 17–18.

Braxton, J. (1991). The influence of graduate department quality on the sanctioning of scientific misconduct. *Journal of Higher Education, 62*, 87–108.

Bulger, R. E. (1994). Toward a statement of the principles underlying responsible conduct in biomedical research. *Academic Medicine, 69*(2), 102–106.

Resnick, D. M. (1993). *Professional ethics for audiologists and speech-language pathologists*. San Diego: Singular Publishing Group. Conflict of interest, pp. 75–79.

Siegel, H. S. (1991). Ethics in research. *Poultry Science, 70*(2), 271–276.

DEMONSTRATION WITHOUT CONSENT

A videotaped session provided clear demonstration of successful implementation of clinical treatment. Unaware that one child's parent did not sign a statement permitting videotaping of the child's sessions for educational use, a faculty member showed the video to an undergraduate class of speech-language pathology majors. One student recognized the child and told the parents about having seen the child in a video shown in class. The parents filed their objections with the clinic supervisor.

Areas of ASHA's Code of Ethics That May Apply

Principle of Ethics I, Rules I and K

Areas of AAA's Code of Ethics That May Apply

Principle 3, Rule 3a

Possible Solutions

1. Review the procedures for informing parents and adult clients about the educational objectives of a university clinic and for assuring that informed consent is obtained from parents or adult clients for videotaping and observation.
2. Review the procedure for informing students about protecting client confidentiality and obtaining informed consent.

Discussion Questions

1. Why would a student or faculty member carelessly violate client confidentiality?
2. Why would parents object to their child appearing on a teaching demonstration video?
3. Are a program's clinical staff and faculty responsible for assuring client confidentiality?

Background Information

American Speech-Language-Hearing Association. (1994). The protection of rights of people receiving audiology or speech-language pathology services. *Asha, 36*(1), 60–63.

American Speech-Language-Hearing Association. (1994). Professional liability and risk management for the audiology and speech-language pathology
professions. *Asha, 36*(Suppl. 12), 25–38.

Darr, K. (1991). *Ethics in health services management.* Baltimore: Health
Professions Press. Consent, pp. 165–178.

DISCRIMINATION

A student clinician is conducting an interview with a transvestite who seeks
assistance in lowering phonatory pitch. While observing through a one-way
mirror, another student clinician states, "I would never work with a person
like that because that lifestyle is against the teachings in the Bible."

Areas of ASHA's Code of Ethics That May Apply

Principle of Ethics I, Rule C

Areas of AAA's Code of Ethics That May Apply

Principle 1, Rule 1a

Possible Solutions

1. The clinical supervisor informs the clinician that her comment violates the ASHA Code of Ethics and is inappropriate.
2. A study of the ASHA and AAA Codes of Ethics is the primary agen-
   da item at the next clinic meeting.

Discussion Questions

1. Might this clinician be prone toward taking a narrow view of some
   personal factors that sometimes kindle discrimination? Explain your
   point of view.
2. Should a religiously based attitude be allowed to influence professional practices?

Background Information

Garnets, L., Hancock, K. A., Cochran, S. D., Goodchilds, J., & Peplau, L. A.
(1991). Issues in psychotherapy with lesbians and gay men. A survey of
psychologists. *American Psychology, 46*(9), 964–972.

Kass, N. E., Faden, R. R., Fox, R., & Dudley, J. (1992). Homosexual and bisexual men's perceptions of discrimination in health services. *American Journal of Public Health, 82*(9), 1277–1279.

Kelly, C. E. (1992). Bring homophobia out of the closet: Antigay bias within the patient-physician relationship. *Comment in: Pharos, 55*(1), 2–8; Pharos, 55(2), 44–45; Pharos, 55(3), 40.

Platzer, H. (1990). Sexual orientation: Improving care. *Nursing Standard, 4*(38), 38–39.

Platzer, H. (1993). Ethics: Nursing care of gay and lesbian patients. *Nursing Standard, 7*(17), 34–37.

Wiltshire, A. (1995). Not by pitch alone: A view of transsexual vocal rehabilitation. *National Student Speech-Language-Hearing Association Journal, 22*, 53–57.

DISHARMONY AMONG STUDENTS

At a student clinician's first meeting with an adult client, the client indicates that the last student assigned to him did not provide successful treatment. The student replied, "Oh, I'm not surprised, she's a really weak student."

Areas of ASHA's Code of Ethics That May Apply

Principle of Ethics III, Rule D
Principle of Ethics IV, Rule B

Areas of AAA's Code of Ethics That May Apply

Principle 6, Rule 6b
Principle 7, Rule 7b
Principle 8, Rule 8b

Possible Solutions

1. Reprimand the student.
2. Review ASHA's and AAA's Codes of Ethics with the student.
3. Review importance of teamwork and harmonious relationship with colleagues.

Discussion Questions

1. Why might a student make such a statement?
2. How might such a comment from a client be handled?

Background Information

Darr, K. (1991). *Ethics in health services management.* Baltimore: Health Professions Press. Chapter 7, Ethical duties toward the organization, pp. 117–138.

Garrett, T. M., Baillie, H. W., & Garrett, R. (1989). *Health care ethics: Principles and problems.* Englewood Cliffs, NJ: Prentice Hall. Chapter 5, Principles of confidentiality and truthfulness, pp. 96–113.

FAULTY FILE MANAGEMENT

You are a student clinician in a university clinic. Your supervisor has stressed repeatedly that client files may not be taken out of the clinic. Reports are due next week and you notice another student slipping client reports into a personal notebook.

Areas of ASHA's Code of Ethics That May Apply

Principle of Ethics I, Rule I

Areas of AAA's Code of Ethics That May Apply

Principle 3, Rule 3a

Possible Solutions

1. Remind the student that client records are not to be taken out of the clinic in an effort to protect confidentiality and in compliance with standards for accreditation of the university program.
2. Report the incident to the supervisor.

Discussion Questions

1. Have students been adequately informed about the Code of Ethics and the standards for accreditation by the Education Standards Board?
2. Are students given adequate time to prepare reports in the clinical setting?
3. Are students who regularly break the rules of practice in a university clinic high risk for engaging in unethical practices as professionals?
4. How might the supervisor handle this situation?
5. Are student peers hesitant to report such incidents? Will they be hesitant to report instances of professional misconduct as professionals? (Principle IV, Rule G ASHA; Principle 8, rule 8a AAA)

Background Information

Darr, K. (1991). *Ethics in health services management.* Baltimore: Health Professions Press.

Flower, R. M. (1984). *Delivery of speech-language pathology and audiology services.* Baltimore: Williams and Wilkins.

Garrett, T. M., Baillie, H. W., & Garrett, R. M. (1989). *Health care ethics.* Englewood Cliffs, NJ: Prentice Hall.

Silverman, F. H. (1992). *Legal-ethical considerations, restrictions, and obligations for clinicians who treat communicative disorders.* Springfield, IL: Charles C. Thomas.

GRADES OVER CLIENT WELFARE

A student clinician never asks the supervisor questions for fear that the supervisor will view this as a weakness when grading the practicum experience. Furthermore, the student is aware that information available in the library would help another student clinician who is working with a similar type of client. However, the student does not share the information for fear that the other student might get a better grade.

Areas of ASHA's Code of Ethics That May Apply

Principle of Ethics I, Rule B
Principle of Ethics IV

Areas of AAA's Code of Ethics That May Apply

Principle 2, Rules 2a and 2b

Possible Solutions

1. Review ASHA's and AAA's Codes of Ethics at the next clinic meeting.
2. Remind students that primary responsibility is to the clients' welfare.
3. Review the standards for grading the practicum experience.
4. Invite a guest lecturer from a local school- or hospital-based team to discuss the team approach and individual behaviors that contribute to a strong team effort.
5. Discuss ways of opening communication between supervisors and student clinicians.
6. Assign clinical practicum team(s) that involve(s) sharing information and responsibility.

Discussion Questions

1. What are the primary fears/anxieties that student clinicians take to the practicum experience?
2. Do you believe that the student clinician honestly is more concerned about the grade than the quality of services or does it just look that way? Why?
3. How might supervisors prevent this type of behavior before it begins?

Background Information

Cahn, S. M. (1994). Rethinking examination and grades. In P. J. Mackie (Ed.), *Professor's duties: Ethical issues in college teaching* (pp. 171–192). Lanham, MD: Rowman and Littlefield Publishers.

McFarlane, L. A., & Hagler, P. (1993). Teams and teamwork: Academic settings. *Asha, 35*(6), 37–38.

INAPPROPRIATE ATTIRE

A student clinician has repeatedly been warned by the supervisor that torn denim pants and sleeveless knit tops are inappropriate clinic wear. The student appears in this attire to meet a client for the third time.

Areas of ASHA's Code of Ethics That May Apply

Principle of Ethics IV

Areas of AAA's Code of Ethics That May Apply

Principle 7

Possible Solutions

1. Review the clinic's dress code.
2. Review the mandate to uphold the dignity of the profession.
3. Remove the student from the practicum experience.

Discussion Questions

1. What if the student does not have clothing appropriate to the clinical setting? Are there financial limitations to acquiring appropriate clothing?
2. Would it be appropriate for the university clinic to provide a uniform for this student to wear?
3. Do students have the same responsibility to look and act professionally as do practicing professionals?
4. How could this problem have been prevented?

Background Information

Draper, D. J., & Whitfield, J. B. (1976). Survey on professional dress. *Journal of National Student Speech and Hearing Association*, 54–62.

Kucera, K. A., & Nicswiadomy, R. M. (1991). Nursing attire: The public's preference. *Nursing Management, 22*(10), 68–70.

Marino, R. V., Rosenfeld, W., Narula, P., & Karakurum, M. (1991). Impact of pediatricians' attire on children and parents. *Developmental and Behavioral Pediatrics, 12*(2), 98–101.

INAPPROPRIATE CREDENTIAL TO SUPERVISE

You are a student in a speech-language pathology program in which the director has a Ph.D., Certificate of Clinical Competence, and a state license in audiology. This individual has been assigned to supervise a portion of your clinical practicum in speech-language pathology.

Areas of ASHA's Code of Ethics That May Apply

Principle of Ethics III, Rules A, B, and D

Areas of AAA's Code of Ethics That May Apply

Principle 5, Rules 5a and 5c
Principle 6, Rule 6a

Possible Solutions

1. Review with the program director the clinical practicum requirements for ASHA CCC in speech-language pathology.
2. Request clarification from ASHA's Committee on Certification.
3. Express your concern to a supervisor in the program who is certified in speech-language pathology.
4. Drop out of the practicum experience.

Discussion Questions

1. How could the situation affect the student's application for clinical certification in speech-language pathology?
2. Could the program director be uninformed about certification requirements for speech-language pathology?
3. How might faculty and/or supervisory staff deal with the situation? Is it their responsibility?

Background Information

American Speech-Language-Hearing Association. (1992). *Educational Standards Board: Accreditation manual.* Rockville, MD: Author.
American Speech-Language-Hearing Association. (1992). *Membership and certification handbook.* Rockville, MD: Author.
American Speech-Language-Hearing Association. (1994). Clinical practice by certificate holders in the profession in which they are not certified. *Asha, 36*(Suppl. 13), 11–12.

INDEPENDENT REFERRAL BY STUDENT

A student clinician told a parent to take a child to a psychologist for intelligence testing without the supervisor's knowledge.

Areas of ASHA's Code of Ethics That May Apply

Principle of Ethics II, Rules A and B

Areas of AAA's Code of Ethics That May Apply

Principle 2, Rule 2d

Possible Solutions

1. Review limitations of the student's scope of practice and the responsibility of the supervisor.
2. Hold a conference with the supervisor, parent, and student clinician to discuss the referral.

Discussion Questions

1. Why might this happen?
2. How are students informed about the responsibility of the supervisor and the scope of practice limitations of students when in the training process?
3. What suggestions might improve all students' understanding of practice limitations?

Background Information

American Speech-Language-Hearing Association. (1992). *Educational Standards Board: Accreditation manual.* Rockville, MD: Author.

American Speech-Language-Hearing Association. (1994). Supervision of student clinicians. *Asha, 36*(Suppl. 13), 13–14.

American Speech-Language-Hearing Association. (1994). *Membership and certification handbook.* Rockville, MD: Author.

INFLATED GRADING

A clinical supervisor permits regularly ill-prepared graduate students to continue in clinical practicum while complaining about their weaknesses, but assigning grades of A and B.

Areas of ASHA's Code of Ethics That May Apply

Principle of Ethics II, Rules B and E
Principle of Ethics IV, Rule B

Areas of AAA's Code of Ethics That May Apply

Principle 8, Rule 8b

Possible Solutions

1. Discuss this discrepancy with the clinical supervisor.
2. Direct attention toward specific areas of concern.
3. Review criteria for assigning clinical grades.
4. Reassign the clinical supervisor.

Discussion Questions

1. Is this chronic behavior for this supervisor?
2. How have students' weaknesses been documented?
3. Is the supervisor providing appropriate feedback to supervisees?

Background Information

American Speech-Language-Hearing Association (1994). Supervision of student clinicians. *Asha, 36*(Suppl. 13), 13–14.

Anderson, M. (1992). *Impostors in the temple.* New York: Simon and Schuster.

Farmer, S. S. (1989). Assessment in supervision. In S. S. Farmer & J. L. Farmer (Eds.), *Supervision in communication disorders* (pp. 274–312). Columbus, OH: Merrill Publishing Company.

Rassi, J. A. (1987). The uniqueness of audiology supervision. In M. B. Crago & M. Pickering (Eds.), *Supervision in human communication disorders* (pp. 31–49). Boston: Little, Brown.

INFORMATION EXPOSURE

A student has been offered a clinical fellowship position as an audiologist with a rehabilitation facility. The position has excellent salary and fringe benefits, which are detailed in a faxed message to the student. The staff member responsible for receiving and distributing faxed messages provides several people with information about the offer.

Areas of ASHA's Code of Ethics That May Apply

Principle of Ethics I, Rule I

Areas of AAA's Code of Ethics That May Apply

Principle 3, Rule 3a

Possible Solutions

1. Review procedures for confidential information.
2. Reprimand the staff member.

Discussion Questions

1. Why do people have difficulty keeping information confidential?
2. How have fax machines and computers added a new dimension to confidentiality?

Background Information

Darr, K. (1991). *Ethics in health services management.* Baltimore: Health Professions Press.

Flower, R. M. (1984). *Delivery of speech-language pathology and audiology services.* Baltimore: Williams and Wilkins.

Garrett, T. M., Baillie, H. W., & Garrett, R. M. (1989). *Health care ethics.* Englewood Cliffs, NJ: Prentice Hall.

Silverman, F. H. (1992). *Legal-ethical considerations, restrictions, and obligations for clinicians who treat communicative disorders.* Springfield, IL: Charles C. Thomas.

INSUFFICIENT SUPERVISION

You are a speech-language pathology major working to complete the required 350 clinic clock hours. You are not being supervised according to ASHA's standards.

Areas of ASHA's Code of Ethics That May Apply

Principle of Ethics II, Rule D

Areas of AAA's Code of Ethics That May Apply

Principle 2, Rules 2d and 2e

Possible Solutions

1. Request reassignment to another supervisor.
2. Review supervision logs with supervisor.
3. Report situation to director of training program.
4. Do nothing.
5. Request assistance from ASHA's Educational Standards Board and Committee on Certification.

Discussion Questions

1. What if this is typical for this supervisor? What if this is typical for other supervisors in this training program?
2. How can the practice be documented?
3. How would this affect the program's accreditation status?

Background Information

American Speech-Language-Hearing Association. (1994). Supervision of student clinicians. *Asha, 36*(Suppl. 13), 13–14.

American Speech-Language Hearing Association. (1992). *Educational Standards Board: Accreditation manual.* Rockville, MD: Author.

American Speech-Language-Hearing Association. (1994). *American speech-language-hearing association membership and certification handbook.* Rockville, MD: Author.

INTERPROFESSIONAL RELATIONSHIPS

You are in your third graduate class. Although the instructor has given lip service to the current push toward consultative and collaborative speech and language services in school settings, he has continually made negative remarks about classroom teachers and their competence. In this class he has been particularly outspoken and vehement, relating his own difficulties in trying to work with school-based teachers. His comments about teachers have included statements like: "they never listen to *you*"; "you're the language expert, and they don't know *anything* about the subject"; and "they're all just stupid!" You express your concern to your advisor.

Areas of ASHA's Code of Ethics That May Apply

Principle of Ethics III, Rules D and E
Principle of Ethics IV, Rules B and F

Areas of AAA's Code of Ethics That May Apply

Principle 6, Rule 6b
Principle 8, Rule 8b

Possible Solutions

1. Graduate advisor and clinic supervisor meet with instructor and express concerns about negative preparation of students for professional collaboration.
2. Clinic supervisor invites a local school-based teacher–SLP team that effectively collaborates to speak to practicum students.
3. Preschool, elementary, and secondary teachers are invited to speak at clinic meetings about successful teacher–SLP working relationships and ways SLPs can benefit children in improving their instructional and social communication in the school setting.
4. Clinic supervisor, student, and instructor meet together to resolve problem.
5. Student is given a list of readings on collaboration and encouraged to report to a class or clinic meeting on effective practices.

Discussion Questions

1. Were other students concerned about instructor's attitude and comments?
2. Was role playing for preventing problematic teacher–SLP interactions attempted? Were problematic interactions specified?

Background Information

Committee on Language Learning Disorders. (1991). A model for collaborative service delivery for students with language-learning disorders in public schools. *Asha, 33*(Suppl. 5), 44–50.

Based on material from: "Ethical considerations in the practice of speech language pathology" by B. N. Witt, 1994 November, Presentation at the meeting of the American Speech-Language-Hearing Association, New Orleans.

IRRESPONSIBLE MENTOR

You are a new faculty member and are assigned a mentor in a university program. Your mentor never contacts you although you repeatedly attempt to contact the mentor without success.

Areas of ASHA's Code of Ethics That May Apply

Principle of Ethics IV

Areas of AAA's Code of Ethics That May Apply

Principle 7

Possible Solutions

1. Report situation to the director of the mentoring program.
2. Request another mentor.
3. Resign from the mentoring program.

Discussion Questions

1. What course of action would you take and why?
2. How can prospective mentors be evaluated?
3. Explain the organization and development of formal mentoring programs.

Background Information

Blosser, J. (1994). Mentoring in the university clinic. *ASHA special interest divisions: Administration and supervision, 4*(3), 9–12.

Jenuchim, J., & Shapiro, P. (1992). *Women, mentors, and success.* New York: Fawcett Columbia.

Kovach, T. M., & Moore, M. S. (1992). Leaders are born through the mentoring process. *Asha, 29*(1), 33–35, 47.

Madison, J. (1994). The value of mentoring in nursing leadership: A descriptive study. *Nursing Forum, 29*(4), 16–23.

Minghetti, N., Cooper, J., Goldstein, H., Olswarg, L., & Warren, S. (Eds.). (1993). *Research mentorship and training in communicative sciences and disorders: Procedures of a national conference.* Rockville, MD: American Speech-Language-Hearing Association.

Morzinski, J. A., Simpson, D. E., Bower, D. J., & Diehr, S. (1994). Faculty development through formal mentoring. *Academic Medicine, 69*(4), 267–269.

Sands, R. G., Parson, L. A., & Duang, J. (1990). Faculty mentoring in a public university. *Journal of Higher Education, 62,* 174–193.

Slater, S. C. (1993). Mentoring: An enriching experience. *Asha, 30*(4), 55.

Wofford, M., Boysen, A., & Riding, L. (1991). A research mentoring process. *Asha, 28*(9), 39–42.

LICENSED ASSISTANT

You are a graduate speech-language pathology student attending a university in a state where the state licenses speech-language pathology assistants, provided they are accepted and enrolled in a graduate speech-language pathology program and have completed a designated number of clinical practicum hours. These individuals are supervised, but the state requirements for supervision are more liberal than are ASHA's. You accept such a position in compliance with state law but in violation of ASHA's Code of Ethics.

Areas of ASHA's Code of Ethics That May Apply

Principle of Ethics II, Rules A, B, D, and E

Areas of AAA's Code of Ethics That May Apply

Principle 2, Rules 2d and 2e
Principle 5, Rule 5c

Possible Solutions

1. Accept no professional position in speech-language pathology until ready for the Clinical Fellowship Year.
2. Agree to work only in a setting with supervision available in compliance with what ASHA would interpret as adequate and appropriate.

Discussion Questions

1. Why are states and ASHA not always in agreement about training and supervision?
2. Should university professors in accredited training programs write recommendations for students seeking such positions?
3. School districts employing such individuals often ask for the university supervisor to place the student for school practicum in the same unit where he or she works as an assistant. Is this appropriate?

Background Information

American Speech-Language-Hearing Association. (1994). Ethical practice inquiries: State versus ASHA jurisdictions. *Asha, 36*(Suppl. 13), 25.
American Speech-Language-Hearing Association. (1981). Employment and utilization of supportive personnel in audiology and speech-language pathology. *Asha, 23*(3), 166–169.

MISREPRESENTATION OF CREDENTIALS

A beginning student clinician purchases a lab coat and a name tag without consulting the clinical supervisor. The name tag provides the student's name followed by the title, "speech-language pathologist." When confronted by the supervisor, the student replies that he feels his credibility with the parents is important to the desired positive outcome of treatment.

Areas of ASHA's Code of Ethics That May Apply

Principle of Ethics III, Rule A
Principle of Ethics IV, Rule A

Areas of AAA's Code of Ethics That May Apply

Principle 6, Rule 6a

Possible Solutions

1. The clinical supervisor orders the student clinician to discontinue wearing the name tag.
2. The student's clients and/or their parents are fully informed about the student's status in training, the supervisory process, and the credentials held by the supervisor.
3. The clinical supervisor provides an in-depth seminar reviewing ASHA and AAA Codes of Ethics at the next clinic meeting.

Discussion Questions

1. What factors would lead a student clinician to be so poorly informed about the ASHA and AAA Codes of Ethics?
2. Why might a student clinician feel adherence to the ASHA and AAA Codes of Ethics unnecessary? How might such an attitude be avoided?
3. If the student continued wearing the name tag, would that be grounds for removing him from the practicum experience?

Background Information

American Speech-Language-Hearing Association. (1992). *Educational Standards Board: Accreditation manual.* Rockville, MD: Author.

NO AVAILABLE SUPERVISOR

You are assigned to a hospital for clinical practicum. Your supervisor is the only ASHA-certified speech-language pathologist. The supervisor is ill and unable to contact you but tells the hospital administrator that you will see his clients.

Areas of ASHA's Code of Ethics That May Apply

Principle of Ethics II, Rule D
Principle of Ethics IV, Rule A

Areas of AAA's Code of Ethics That May Apply

Principle 2, Rules 2d and 2e
Principle 7, Rule 7b

Possible Solutions

1. Do nothing—that is, see the clients.
2. Call the university supervisor.
3. Leave the hospital after informing the administrator.

Discussion Questions

1. Why would a hospital supervisor believe the student clinician could see his clients while he was ill?
2. What would you do if this happened to you?
3. What could be done to prevent this situation?
4. What should the university supervisor do?

Background Information

American Speech-Language-Hearing Association. (1994). Supervision of student clinicians. *Asha, 36*(Suppl. 13), 13–14.

American Speech-Language Hearing Association. (1992). *Educational Standards Board: Accreditation manual*. Rockville, MD: Author.

American Speech-Language-Hearing Association. (1994). *American speech-language hearing association membership and certification handbook*. Rockville, MD: Author.

OFF-SITE PRACTICUM COMPLIANCE

You are the university supervisor assigned to coordinate off-site practicae. Three students assigned to a hospital for clinical practicum report concerns related to lack of supervision, supervisors not being on site, admission criteria for speech-language treatment, and inadequate time allocation for audiology assessment. These concerns have been documented, and although discussed with the hospital speech-language pathology and audiology supervisors, they continue to be problems.

Areas of ASHA's Code of Ethics That May Apply

Principle of Ethics I
Principle of Ethics II, Rule D
Principle of Ethics IV, Rule A

Areas of AAA's Code of Ethics That May Apply

Principle 2, Rule 2e

Possible Solutions

1. Do nothing.
2. Let the students complete the practicum, but not assign students to this site in the future.
3. Discuss the concerns and the possible solution(s) if the problem(s) continue with the hospital supervisors.
4. Discuss the situation with the hospital administrator.
5. Discontinue the practicum immediately.
6. Refer the issues to the hospital ethics committee.
7. Utilize logs for recording clinical clock hours that include information about "percentage of supervision."

Discussion Questions

1. Would it matter if this practice is typical for this hospital?
2. How could this be avoided in the future?
3. How can similar problems be prevented at other off-site practicum facilities?

Background Information

American Speech-Language-Hearing Association. (1985). Clinical supervision position statement. *Asha, 27*(6), 57–60.
American Speech-Language-Hearing Association. (1994). *American Speech-Language-Hearing Association membership and certification handbook.* Rockville, MD: Author.

PAID CLINICAL PRACTICUM

A student clinician is employed by an area school district as a bachelor's level speech-language therapy assistant. The school district's Supervisor of Speech-Language Services requests that the student be placed in her work therapy unit for the required practicum experience. The university supervisor is assured that the supervising speech-language pathologist with CCC-SLP will be on-site and supervising in compliance with ASHA certification requirements. After 3 weeks in the experience, the university supervisor discovers that the student is being paid a regular salary and that the supervisor is rarely on-site.

Areas of ASHA's Code of Ethics That May Apply

Principle of Ethics I
Principle of Ethics II, Rules A, B, D, and E
Principle of Ethics IV, Rule B

Areas of AAA's Code of Ethics That May Apply

Principle 2, Rule 2d

Possible Solutions

1. Move the student to a different placement in a different school district.
2. Review with the supervisor of record the ultimate supervisory responsibility for the services rendered by the student.
3. Discuss the original agreement and current practice with the school district's Supervisor of Speech-Language Services.

Discussion Questions

1. Would it have mattered if the original agreement was violated without the district's Supervisor of Speech-Language Services knowledge? Who is ultimately responsible for the situation?
2. Why do you think the university supervisor was willing to place the student according to the request by the district's representative?
3. Should the student receive practicum hours for the 3 weeks completed under these conditions?

4. Was the student responsible for reporting the situation?

5. For what reason(s) might the student not have reported the situation?

6. Does a paid practicum experience constitute condition(s) for a conflict of interest?

Background Information

Anderson, J. L. (1988). *The supervisory process in speech-language pathology and audiology*. Boston: Little, Brown, and Company.

Dowling, S. (1992). *Implementing the supervisory process: Theory and practice*. Englewood Cliffs, NJ: Prentice Hall.

Farmer, S. S., & Farmer, J. L. (1989). *Supervision in communication disorders*. Columbus, OH: Merrill Publishing Co.

O'Toole, T. (1995, February). *LC 50-94 Pay for Practicum*. (Available from the American Speech-Language-Hearing Association, 10801 Rockville Pike, Rockville, MD 20852.)

PLAGIARIZING A DIAGNOSTIC REPORT

A student enrolled in clinical practicum has had a diagnostic report returned for the second time with only the recommendation to revise the report. On her request, you have provided your report on the same client. Your report had been approved, graded, and returned by the supervisor. The student copied your report and turned it in to the supervisor. The supervisor calls both of you in for questioning.

Areas of ASHA's Code of Ethics That May Apply

Principle of Ethics I, Rules H and I
Principle of Ethics II

Areas of AAA's Code of Ethics That May Apply

Principle 3, Rule 3a
Principle 5, Rule 5d

Possible Solutions

1. Review the requirements for successful completion of the practicum experience.

2. Discuss the difference between teamwork and plagiarism.
3. Report the incident to the Dean of Students.
4. Review the university definition of scholastic dishonesty.

Discussion Questions

1. Were both students to blame in this incident? Explain.
2. How might plagiarism in practicum ultimately impact the quality of client care?
3. Did the supervisor provide adequate feedback to the struggling student?
4. Is the practicum experience under the same regulations as lecture classes in terms of scholastic honesty?

Background Information

Armstrong, J. D. (1993). Plagiarism: What is it, whom does it affect, and how does one deal with it? *American Journal of Radiology, 161*, 479–484.
Hoekema, D. A. (1994). *Campus rules and moral community*. Lanham, MD: Rowman and Littlefield Publishers.

POOR PROFESSIONAL RELATIONSHIPS

At an open house for area students and practicing speech-language pathologists, a student is asked by a supervisor what employment area interests the student. The student is interested in the public schools. The supervisor responds, "That's such a waste of time. You are too smart for the public schools."

Areas of ASHA's Code of Ethics That May Apply

Principle of Ethics IV

Areas of AAA's Code of Ethics That May Apply

Principle 7, Rule 7a

Possible Solutions

1. Discuss the negative attitude with the supervisor.
2. Pretend the statement was not made.
3. Identify positive features of employment in the public schools.

Discussion Questions

1. If public school clinicians overheard this comment, how do you think they might feel?
2. What would be an appropriate response to this comment?
3. Why are there negative attitudes about speech-language services in the schools?

Background Information

Hall, S., Larrigan, L. B., & Madison, C. L. (1991). A comparison of speech-language pathologists in rural and urban school districts in the state of Washington. *Language Speech Hearing Services Schools, 22*(4), 204–210.

Pezzei, C., & Oratio, A. R. (1991). A multivariate analysis of the job satisfaction of public school speech-language pathologists. *Language Speech Hearing Services Schools, 22*(3), 139–146.

Sanger, D. D., Hux, K., & Griess, K. (1995). Educators' opinions about speech-language pathology services in schools. *Language Speech Hearing Services Schools, 26*(1), 75–83.

Saricks, M. C. B. (1989). School services and communication disorders. *Asha, 32*(6), 79–80.

Simon, C. (1991). A profession in transition: Thoughts on the speech-language pathologist as a school language specialist. *National Student Speech Language Hearing Association Journal, 18*, 26–33.

Tomes, L., & Sanger, D. D. (1986). Attitudes of interdisciplinary team members toward speech-language services in public schools. *Language Speech Hearing Services Schools, 17*(3), 230–240.

SALARY COMPRESSION

At a meeting of program directors in speech-language pathology and audiology, the impact of personnel shortages on entry-level salaries and salary compression are discussed. One of the program directors suggests that salary compression should not be recognized or discussed. His words are "Don't tell them; ignore it."

Areas of ASHA's Code of Ethics That May Apply

Principle of Ethics III, Rule B
Principle of Ethics IV, Rule B
Principle of Ethics IV, Rule D

Areas of AAA's Code of Ethics That May Apply

Principle 6, Rule 6b
Principle 7, Rule 7b

Possible Solutions

1. Periodic review and adjustment of salaries
2. Do nothing because salary compression exists in all areas.

Discussion Questions

1. How prevalent is salary compression in speech-language pathology and audiology training programs?
2. What can be done to reduce or eliminate salary inequities?
3. Are long-term faculty members typically aware of salary compression?
4. Why does salary compression exist?
5. How serious are salary inequities?
6. Does periodic evaluation and review for merit reduce salary compression?
7. What is the impact of salary compression on faculty productivity?

Background Information

McCulley, W. L., & Downey, R. G. (1993). Salary compression in faculty salaries: Identification of a suppressor effect. *Education and Psychological Measurement, 53,* 79–86.
Leatherman, C. (1995). Outpacing inflation. *The Chronicle of Higher Education,* A20–A26.

Seldin, P. (1988). *Evaluating and developing administrative performance.* San Francisco: Jossey-Bass.

Snyder. K. K. (1992). Diagnosing and dealing with salary compression. *Research in Higher Education, 33*(1), 113–124.

Tesch, B. J., Wood, H. M., Helwig, A. L., & Nattinger, A. B. (1995). Promotion of women physicians in academic medicine: Glass ceiling or sticky floor. *Journal of American Medical Association, 273*(13), 1022–1025.

SELF-REFERRALS

A speech-language pathologist who is a faculty member in a communication sciences and disorders program with an on-site speech and hearing clinic also has a private practice. The speech-language pathologist instructs the clinic secretary to schedule only the clients unable to pay for speech-language evaluations. The secretary is further instructed to refer clients who have insurance or ability to pay to the speech-language pathologist's private practice.

Areas of ASHA's Code of Ethics That May Apply

Principle of Ethics III, Rule B

Possible Solutions

1. Provide the speech-language pathologist with information about self-referrals and conflicts of professional interest, indicating that "individuals who work in one professional setting should not refer clients exclusively to themselves in another professional setting" (ASHA, 1994, p. 8).
2. Ignore the situation.
3. Inform the department head and/or college dean about the situation.
4. Approach the speech-language pathologist and request that the speech-language pathologist discontinue this referral system.
5. Instruct the secretary that referral must not be made to the speech-language pathologist's private practice.

Discussion Questions

1. What are the ramifications of the continuation of this practice?
2. What if you say nothing and some other professional reports the situation?

3. What if the speech-language pathologist is told to stop these self-referrals and disregards this request?
4. Does the speech-language pathologist's university have a faculty practice plan? If so, is faculty practice outside the plan prohibited?
5. To what extent might personal financial gains be motivating the faculty member?

Background Information

American Speech-Language-Hearing Association. (1994). Conflicts of professional interest. *Asha, 36*(Suppl. 13), 7–8.
American Speech-Language-Hearing Association. (1994). Drawing cases for private practice from primary place of employment. *Asha, 36*(Suppl. 13), 21.

SELF-SERVING AUTHORITY

An audiologist who is an associate professor at a university is currently chairing the promotions committee. This audiologist is concurrently considered for promotion and is promoted from associate to full professor.

Areas of ASHA's Code of Ethics That May Apply

Principle of Ethics III, Rule E
Principle of Ethics IV, Rule D

Areas of AAA's Code of Ethics That May Apply

Principle 6, Rule 6b
Principle 7, Rule 7b

Possible Solutions

1. Report the situation to the university president.
2. Notify accrediting agency(s).
3. If you are a member of the committee, resign.
4. Contact the American Association of University Professors.
5. Develop guidelines for serving on the promotions committee.

Discussion Questions

1. Should data supporting the chair's promotion be considered in evaluating the ethics of such a situation?
2. Would the perceptions of committee members about the promotion matter?
3. What would have been the difference if faculty members had concurred with the promotion? If they had not agreed? If there was no faculty reaction?
4. Might the committee have not recommended the promotion? What would have been the basis for this?

Background Information

Centra, J. A. (1980). *Determining faculty effectiveness*. San Francisco: Jossey-Bass Publishers.

Markie, P. J. (1994). *Professor's duties: Ethical issues in college teaching*. Lanham, MD: Rowman and Littlefield Publishers.

Miller, R. I. (1987). *Evaluating faculty for promotion and tenure*. San Francisco: Jossey-Bass Publishers.

STUDENT CLINICIAN COMPLAINTS

A student clinician comes to you to complain about another supervisor's shortcomings in grading and supervision.

Areas of ASHA's Code of Ethics That May Apply

Principle of Ethics IV, Rule D

Areas of AAA's Code of Ethics That May Apply

Principle 6, Rule 6b

Possible Solutions

1. Alert student clinicians about appropriate procedures for complaints during the first week of the semester, preferably in the clinic handbook for students.

2. Do not listen to complaints about another supervisor. Send the student clinician back to original supervisor.
3. If this fails, the student should see the clinic director.
4. Next step is see the department head.
5. Next step is filing a formal grievance.

Discussion Questions

1. Under what circumstances should a student clinician go directly to the clinic director?
2. What data are needed to file a formal grievance?

Background Information

American Speech-Language-Hearing Association. (1985). Clinical supervision statement. *Asha, 27*(6), 57–60.

Gerstman, H. L. (1977). Supervisory relationships: Experiences in dynamic communication. *Asha, 19*(8), 527–529.

Harris, H. F., Lundington, J. R., Ringwalt, S. S., Ballard, D. D., Hooper, C. R., Buoyer, F. G., & Price, K. R. (1991–1992). Involving the student in the supervisory process. *National Student Speech-Language-Hearing Association Journal, 19*, 109–118.

STUDENT IN PRIVATE PRACTICE

You are a student clinician whose client made exceptional progress during the fall semester. The child's grateful parents fear that the child will not progress over the long winter holiday without continued treatment. They ask you to continue working with the client for 2 hours a week at $15 an hour.

Areas of ASHA's Code of Ethics That May Apply

Principle of Ethics II, Rules A and B

Areas of AAA's Code of Ethics That May Apply

Principle 2, Rules 2a, 2d, and 2e

Possible Solutions

1. Provide the parents with activities to do with the child over the holidays.
2. Conduct practice activities while hired as a baby sitter at the going rate for that service.
3. Encourage the parents to enroll the child with a certified and licensed speech-language pathologist in private practice.

Discussion Questions

1. Is it appropriate for a student clinician to conduct follow-up activities without supervision?
2. If yes, under what circumstances? If no, why?
3. Who is responsible for explaining the role of a student clinician's practice limitations to parents?

Background Information

Reichert, A. M., & Caruso, A. J. (1990–1991). Ethical standards in the university clinic: A student perspective. *National Student Speech-Language-Hearing Association, 18*, 137–141.

TIME COMMITMENT CONFLICT

Because a student clinician works in a restaurant during every available non-class hour in the day, he does not sign up for regular conferences with the supervisor. On being reminded about the conference requirement, the student replies, "You will have to extend your conference hours to times I am not working or I cannot schedule conferences with you."

Areas of ASHA's Code of Ethics That May Apply

Principle of Ethics I, Rule B
Principle of Ethics II, Rule D
Principle of Ethics IV

Areas of AAA's Code of Ethics That May Apply

Principle 2, Rules 2a and 2f
Principle 7

Possible Solutions

1. Inform the student about a clinician's responsibility to hold paramount the welfare of persons served professionally.
2. Consider either reducing work hours or dropping clinic until more time can be given to the clinical experience.
3. Review college/university policy about student academic and employment workloads.

Discussion Questions

1. Can a student with such a schedule receive maximum training from the practicum experience?
2. Do financial needs outweigh meeting of educational objectives of students?
3. Are there solutions for this dilemma?
4. What responsibility do students have to the welfare of their future clients?

Background Information

Gerstman, H. L. (1977). Supervising relationships: Experience in dynamic communication. *Asha, 19*(8), 527–529.

TREATMENT EFFICACY VS. STUDENT TRAINING

You are a graduate student clinician working with an adult client with cerebral palsy in the university clinic. On your careful review of the client's records of very limited improvement over the past three semesters of treatment, you question the efficacy of continued therapy. The supervisor responds that the client enjoys therapy and wants to continue. Furthermore, the client provides excellent training for students who need to complete practicum hours with adult clients.

Areas of ASHA's Code of Ethics That May Apply

Principle of Ethics I, Rule E

Areas of AAA's Code of Ethics That May Apply

Principle 4, Rule 4a

Possible Solutions

1. Leave the decision to continue treatment with the client after fully informing him about probable limited improvement.
2. Do not charge for the treatment.
3. Dismiss the client.

Discussion Questions

1. Is it appropriate to continue working with a client simply because he or she is unusual enough to offer "good practice" for students?
2. Would the client better benefit from another program, such as an adult activities program for socialization and leisure time activities?
3. What might be the client's real motive or reason for continuing the treatment?
4. Does the therapy funding source have impact on continuation of treatment?

Background Information

American Speech-Language-Hearing Association. (1993). Preferred practice patterns for the profession of speech-language pathology and audiology. *Asha, 35*(Suppl. 3), 83–84.

UNCERTIFIED SUPERVISOR

You are a student enrolled in practicum. The individual directly supervising you is not certified. Your hour logs are being signed by a certified supervisor who is not assigned to supervise you. When you ask the program director about the situation, you are told that it makes no difference who signs your hour logs, as long as that supervisor is certified.

Areas of ASHA's Code of Ethics That May Apply

Principle of Ethics II, Rules A, B, D, and E
Principle of Ethics IV, Rules A and B

Areas of AAA's Code of Ethics That May Apply

Principle 2, Rule 2d
Principle 6, Rule 6a

Possible Solutions

1. Review the clinical practicum requirements for ASHA CCCs in speech-language pathology with the program administrator.
2. Request clarification from ASHA's Committee on Certification.
3. Express your concern to a certified supervisor in the program.
4. Drop out of the practicum experience.

Discussion Questions

1. Is the program out of compliance with Educational Standards Board Accreditation and with the standards for certification?
2. What condition(s) might cause a program to hire an uncertified supervisor?
3. Whose responsibility is it to correct this problem?
4. Is the program director uninformed about certification requirements for speech-language pathology?
5. How would the situation later effect the student's application for clinical certification in speech-language pathology?

Background Information

American Speech-Language-Hearing Association. (1994). *Membership and certification handbook*. Rockville, MD: Author.
American Speech-Language-Hearing Association. (1994). Supervision of student clinicians. *Asha, 36*(Suppl. 13), 13–14.

UNFAIR AND INSUFFICIENT SUPERVISION

You are a speech-language pathology graduate student working to complete the required 350 clinic clock hours for ASHA CCC and are scheduled to graduate at the end of the current semester. At the middle of the semester all clinical paper work was up-to-date. Your supervisor had not observed any treatment sessions since the initial session, but gave "blind advice" about procedures. You have repeatedly told your supervisor that these treatment procedures are "not working." At the end of the semester, your supervisor observed the final treatment session. The supervisor enters the treatment room and questions the procedures that are being used. Your clinic grade is based on this final session.

Areas of ASHA's Code of Ethics That May Apply

Principle of Ethics II, Rule D
Principle of Ethics IV, Rule B

Possible Solutions

1. Meet with the supervisor and discuss concerns about lack of supervision.
2. Request that the client be assigned to another supervisor.
3. Report the situation to director of training program.
4. Say nothing and pretend the events did not happen.
5. Document the situation.

Discussion Questions

1. What if the supervisor continues this supervisory practice?
2. What if you report the supervisor to someone and you have to repeat all of the treatment hours that were not properly supervised?
3. What could be the result if this is typical of this supervisor or of other supervisors in the training program?
4. What recourse is available to the student clinician?
5. How can the problem be documented?

Background Information

American Speech-Language-Hearing Association. (1994). Supervision of student clinicians. *Asha, 36*(Suppl. 13), 13–14.

American Speech-Language-Hearing Association. (1992). *Educational Standards Board: Accreditation manual.* Rockville, MD: Author.

American Speech-Language-Hearing Association. (1994). *American Speech-Language-Hearing Association membership and certification handbook.* Rockville, MD: Author.

Culatta, R. (1992). Where has the master clinician gone? Progress v. content. *Asha, 34*(8), 49–50.

Culatta, R., & Helmick, J. W. (1981). Clinical supervision: The state of the art, Part II: Clinical session, supervisory session, and evaluation of supervisory performance. *Asha, 23*(1), 21–27.

Hagler, P., & Casey, P. L. (1990). Games supervisors play in clinical supervision. *Asha, 32*(2), 53–56.

Hegde, M. N., & Davis, D. (1995). *Clinical methods and practicum in speech-language pathology.* San Diego: Singular Publishing Group. Chapter 4, The supervisor and the student clinician, pp. 81–98.

Ulrich, S. R. (1992). Issues for academia. *Asha, 34*(8), 51–52.

Based on material from: "Ethical considerations in the practice of speech-language pathology" by G. Easterly, A. Tapp, & C. Yager, 1994 November, Presentation at the meeting of the American Speech-Language-Hearing Association, New Orleans.

UNFAIR TREATMENT OF SUPERVISEE

You are a speech-language pathology graduate student completing the required 350 clinic clock hours for ASHA CCC. You have accumulated 300 clinic clock hours so far with all A's in your practicum classes. At midterm your clinic practicum grade was A, but your clinic supervisor continually identifies your weaknesses in diagnosis and treatment. Occasionally you have been belittled and humiliated by this supervisor in front of classmates and other supervisors.

Areas of ASHA's Code of Ethics That May Apply

Principle of Ethics I, Rule I
Principle of Ethics IV, Rule D

Possible Solutions

1. Confer directly with the supervisor about the situation.
2. Request a change of supervisors.

3. Report the supervisor to the director of training program.
4. Document this supervisor's behavior.
5. Student rating of the supervisor should reflect this situation.

Discussion Questions

1. What if other students have had similar experiences with this supervisor?
2. How can the matter be addressed and protect confidential information?

Background Information

Anderson, M. (1992). *Impostors in the temple.* New York: Simon and Schuster.

Gerstman, H. L. (1977). Supervisory relationships: Experiences in dynamic communication. *Asha, 19*(8), 527–529.

Hagler, P., & Casey, P. L. (1990). Games supervisors play in clinical supervision. *Asha, 32*(2), 53–55.

UNLICENSED FACULTY PRACTICE PLAN MEMBER

An ASHA certified speech-language pathologist is a member of a faculty practice plan at the university where she has been employed as an associate professor for 5 years. A faculty practice plan is an arrangement for billing, collecting, and distributing clinical service income to faculty for either direct provision of clinical service or supervision of graduate students. The state in which this speech-language pathologist is employed has mandatory licensure for all speech-language pathologists; however, this speech-language pathologist is not licensed.

Areas of ASHA's Code of Ethics That May Apply

Principle of Ethics IV, Rule B

Possible Solutions

1. Request clarification from ASHA's Ethical Practice Board and state licensure board.
2. Inform the individual of the appearance of impropriety.
3. The individual withdraws from faculty practice plan.

4. The individual obtains state license and maintains membership in faculty practice plan.
5. Review the situation with university administrators.

Discussion Questions

1. What are the possible consequences of this situation?
2. How could this situation be avoided?
3. Which is of more concern in this situation—an apparent ethical violation or the appearance of an ethical violation?
4. What are the legal ramifications for the faculty member and the program?

Background Information

American Speech-Language-Hearing Association. (1994). Ethical practice inquiries: State versus ASHA jurisdictions. *Asha, 36*(Suppl. 13), 25.

Chicadonz, G. H. (1987). Faculty practice. *Annual Review of Nursing Research, 5,* 137–151.

Cunningham, D. R., Baker, B. M., Steckol, K. F., & Windmill, I. M. (1989). The unification model: Ten years of faculty private practice. *Asha, 31*(9), 87–89.

Langford, T. L. (1987). The politics of faculty practice: The dean's role. *Nursing Outlook, 35*(4), 178–181.

O'Hollaren, M. T., et al. (1992). A model for faculty practice teaching clinics developed at the Oregon Health Sciences University. *Academic Medicine, 67*(1), 51–53.

Shnorhokian, H. I., & Zullo, T. G. (1993). A survey of faculty practice plans in United States and Canadian dental schools. *Journal of Dental Education, 57*(4), 318–320.

UNPREPARED FOR TREATMENT

A student clinician repeatedly turns in treatment plans that are deemed unsatisfactory by the supervisor. The student also repeatedly does not meet with the supervisor nor does the student modify a treatment plan prior to meeting with the client.

Areas of ASHA's Code of Ethics That May Apply

Principle of Ethics I, Rule A
Principle of Ethics II, Rules D and E

Areas of AAA's Code of Ethics That May Apply

Principle 2, Rule 2d

Possible Solutions

1. Review the procedure for lesson plan approval prior to providing treatment.
2. The supervisor provides treatment when lesson plans are not approved.

Discussion Questions

1. Are there possible scheduling problems that could cause a student to be unable to meet with a supervisor between the time the student receives an unapproved lesson plan and the time the client is scheduled?
2. Would it matter if the supervisor had been available for conferences with the student to discuss plans for the upcoming week(s)? Should students schedule such conferences with supervisors?
3. Should students receive clinical hours for treatment administered without approved lesson plans?
4. Who is ultimately responsible for the quality of treatment in this situation?
5. Should students be allowed to administer treatment using unapproved lesson plans?

Background Information

American Speech-Language-Hearing Association. (1994). Supervision of student clinicians. *Asha, 36*(Suppl. 13), 13–14.

C H A P T E R 3

CLINICAL CASE STUDIES

Several issues confront speech-language pathologists and audiologists involved in clinical practice. Issues included in this chapter are summarized in Table 3–1.

TABLE 3–1. Summary of Clinical Case Studies

Page	Title and Topic	Concepts and Issue
77	Advertising and Availability of Services	Overload; compromised quality of services
78	Amplification for Client in Remote Area	Services by correspondence
79	Audiologist's Advertisement Discrediting Hearing Aid Dealers	Blatant misrepresentation in advertising
80	Audiology Practice Outside Scope of Practice	Untrained to provide service

(continued)

TABLE 3–1. *(continued)*

Page	Title and Topic	Concepts and Issue
82	Audiology Services in a Nursing Home	Inadequate facility and diagnosis
83	Auditory Integration Training	Experimental treatment
84	Billing Improprieties	Misrepresentation of services for reimbursement; informing Ethical Practice Board
85	Burnout and Alcoholism	Substance abuse
86	Cerumen Management	Untrained to provide service
87	Child Abuse by an Audiologist	Off-duty behaviors
88	Collaborative Service	Inaccurate information; discrimination
90	Confidentiality and Telephone Message	Inadvertent dissemination of clinical information
91	Continuing Education	Professional development
92	Demarketing	Welfare of client; conflict of interest
93	Dysphagia Training	Clinical competence
94	Dysphagia Treatment	Welfare of client; clinical competence
95	Electronic Breach of Confidentiality	Failure to protect confidential information
96	Expiration of Financial Benefits	Welfare of client
98	Fabricating Evaluation Results	Inadequate records; charging for services not rendered
99	Facilitated Communication	Effectiveness of services

TABLE 3–1. *(continued)*

Page	Title and Topic	Concepts and Issue
100	Failure To Refer	Clinical competency; resource utilization
101	Falsifying Credentials	Misrepresentation of credentials
102	Falsifying Records	Dishonesty
103	Financial Conflict of Interest	Personal financial gain
104	Guaranteed Results	Welfare of client; responsibilities to profession
106	Hearing Screening	Failure to screen hearing; welfare of client
107	HIV Issues—1	Discrimination in delivery of services
108	HIV Issues—2	Discrimination in delivery of services
109	Inadequate Bilingual Services	Welfare of bilingual clients
110	Inadequate CF Supervision	Client welfare
111	Inadequate Record Keeping	Documentation of services
112	Incompetency	Not certified or licensed to provide audiologic services
113	Indirect Evaluation	Treating by correspondence; harmonious relationship with colleague
115	Lack of Adherence to Universal Precautions	Client and clinician welfare
116	Lack of Independent Professional Judgment	Welfare of client; independent judgment

(continued)

TABLE 3–1. *(continued)*

Page	Title and Topic	Concepts and Issue
117	Medicaid	Misrepresentation and charging for services not rendered
118	Misleading the Public	Misinformation about effects of services; marketing services violates professional standards
120	Mistaken Diagnosis of Hearing Impairment	Conflict of interest
121	Negative Prognosis	Effectiveness of services; unreasonable expectations
122	Negligent Clinical Fellowship Supervisor	Irresponsible supervisor
123	Noncompliance With IEP	Recruitment and retention of speech-language pathologists
124	Patient Competency and Decision Making	Rights of patients
125	Poor Treatment Facilities	Environmentally unsound treatment facility
126	Poor Professional Relations	Misrepresentation; conflict of interest
127	Poor Prognosis	Continuation of treatment without improvement
128	Practice Outside Scope of Competence	Lack of training and experience
129	Professional Disharmony	Client welfare; documentation
130	Psychogenic Hearing Loss	Incorrect diagnosis
131	Quotas—1	Welfare of client; conflict of interest
132	Quotas—2	Welfare of client; conflict of interest
133	Refusal to Refer	Welfare of client; clinician competency

TABLE 3–1. *(continued)*

Page	Title and Topic	Concepts and Issue
134	Refusal to Treat Medicare/ Medicaid Clients	Discrimination in service delivery
135	Reporting Child Abuse	Welfare of client
136	Self-Consultation	Charging for services that are nondocumentable
137	Speech-Language Pathology Practice Outside Scope of Practice	Inadequate preparation
138	Speech Therapy Assistant	Welfare of client; delegating services
139	Support Personnel	Inappropriate supervision; delegating services
140	Unfunded Independent Judgment	Clinician versus insurance funding
141	Unsatisfactory Clinical Fellow	Client welfare
143	Untreated Hearing Loss in a Child	Client welfare

ADVERTISING AND AVAILABILITY OF SERVICES

A new rehabilitation unit opens in a city where there is strong competition from established rehabilitation hospitals. The new program is creatively and effectively advertised and marketed. More referrals than the speech-language pathologists can handle are accepted. Advertised quality of services is thus compromised.

Areas of ASHA's Code of Ethics That May Apply

Principle of Ethics I, Rules A and B
Principle of Ethics III, Rule E

Possible Solutions

1. Hire additional speech-language pathologists.
2. Limit acceptance of referrals according to space in the caseload.
3. Decrease advertising.

Discussion Questions

1. Are clients being accepted for occupational therapy and physical therapy in need of speech-language services, but not receiving these services because of lack of space in the caseload? If so, is this appropriate?
2. If not appropriate, would it be better to provide some services, though inadequate, rather than none at all?
3. Could some of the advertising budget be redirected to funding in areas of need?

Background Information

American Speech-Language-Hearing Association. (1994). Public announcements and public statements. *Asha, 36*(Suppl. 13), 19–20.

AMPLIFICATION FOR CLIENT IN REMOTE AREA

A client writes to an audiologist explaining that she is having considerable difficulty hearing in a variety of situations. She lives in a remote area about 250 miles from any available services. She explains that it is not possible for her to travel for testing. It is also impossible for the audiologist to arrange to provide services in her area. The audiologist sends her a detailed questionnaire to obtain information about medical conditions, the range of her hearing, and areas of difficulty.

Areas of ASHA's Code of Ethics That May Apply

Principle of Ethics I, Rule G

Areas of AAA's Code of Ethics That May Apply

Principle 2, Rule 2c

Possible Solutions

1. Insist that the client travel to the facility for at least one testing session.
2. Refer the client to a hearing aid dealer who makes home visits.
3. Go to the client's home to perform testing to the extent possible.
4. Inform the client that services cannot be provided solely on a correspondence basis.
5. Seek to locate an audiologist closer to the client who may be in a better position to provide services.

Discussion Questions

1. Can the client be helped by services provided solely by correspondence?
2. What is the professional's obligation to serve someone who needs assistance and may not be able to obtain it directly?
3. What obligations do professionals have in making referral to another resource?

Background Information

American Speech-Language-Hearing Association. (1988, March). The delivery of speech-language pathology and audiology services in home care. *Asha, 30*, 77–79.

Rupp, R. R., Vaughn, G. R., & Lightfoot, R. K. (1984). Nontraditional 'aids' to hearing: Assistive listening devices. *Geriatrics, 39*(3), 55–56, 61–67, 71–73.

Vaughn, G. R. (1976). Tel-communicology health care delivery system for persons with communication disorders. *Asha, 18*(1), 13–17.

Vaughn, G. R. (1983). Assistive listening devices and systems (ALDS) enhance the lifestyles of hearing impaired persons. *American Journal of Otolaryngology, 4* (Suppl. 9), 101–106.

Vaughn, G. R. (1983). Assistive listening devices—Part II: Large area sound systems. *Asha, 25*(3), 25–30.

Vaughn, G. R., Lightfoot, R. K., & Gibbs, S. D. (1983). Assistive listening devices—Part III: SPACE. *Asha, 25*(3), 33–39, 41–42, 44–46.

AUDIOLOGIST'S ADVERTISEMENT DISCREDITING HEARING AID DEALERS

An audiologist places an advertisement in a local newspaper stating that the average hearing aid dealer is not always qualified to do all the tests and evaluations crucial to a person's hearing. He further states, "success with hearing aids is 13 times greater when they are provided by an audiologist."

Area's of ASHA's Code of Ethics That May Apply

Principle of Ethics III, Rules D and E
Principle of Ethics IV, Rule D

Areas of AAA's Code of Ethics That May Apply

Principle 5
Principle 6, Rule 6b
Principle 7, Rule 7a

Possible Solutions

1. Print a retraction.
2. Discontinue advertisements of this type.

Discussion Questions

1. What if there is documentation for these claims?
2. Can this kind of advertising backfire?
3. Does this violate federal Food and Drug Administration policies?

Background Information

Helmick, J. W. (1994). Ethics and the profession of audiology. *Seminars in Hearing, 15*(3). 190–198.

Clark, J. G. (1993). Audiology's marketing dilemma: One possible solution. *Audiology Today, 5*(5), 23–24.

Resnick, D. M. (1992). Issues in ethics: Balancing the ethics of a profession and a business. *Audiology Today, 4*(2), 18–20.

AUDIOLOGY PRACTICE OUTSIDE SCOPE OF PRACTICE

An audiologist who graduated 20 years ago has recently changed jobs. He was not trained to do electrophysiologic testing and his previous job did not require it. In his new job in an otoneurologist's office, he is expected to do intraoperative monitoring.

Areas of ASHA's Code of Ethics That May Apply

Principle of Ethics I, Rule A
Principle of Ethics II, Rules B and E

Areas of AAA's Code of Ethics That May Apply

Principle 2, Rule 2f

Possible Solutions

1. Explain to the new employer before taking the job that additional training is needed in this area.
2. Enroll in a workshop, course and/or practicum experience to develop skills in this area.
3. Say nothing and attempt to perform intraoperative monitoring.
4. Turn down the job.

Discussion Questions

1. What if the audiologist loses his chance for this job by admitting his deficiencies?
2. Who will bear the expense of additional training, the audiologist or the new employer?
3. What if a client is injured because of the audiologist's inexperience?

Background Information

American Speech-Language-Hearing Association. (1990). Scope of practice. *Asha, 32*(Suppl. 2), 1.
American Speech-Language-Hearing Association. (1992). Neurophysiologic intraoperative monitoring. *Asha, 34*(Suppl. 7), 34–36.
Dennis, J. M. (1992). Neurophysiological intraoperative monitoring. *American Journal of Audiology, 2*, 44–56.

AUDIOLOGY SERVICES IN A NURSING HOME

An audiologist is providing services in a nursing home. The residents, for the most part, cannot be tested in a sound-treated booth. It is either physically impossible for them to go to a facility with a booth or they cannot afford the transportation. Several residents are fitted with hearing aids on the basis of results obtained in the nursing home.

Areas of ASHA's Code of Ethics That May Apply

Principle of Ethics I, Rules A, B, C, and E
Principle of Ethics III

Areas of AAA's Code of Ethics That May Apply

Principle 1, Rule 1a
Principle 2, Rules 2b and 2c
Principle 4, Rule 4a

Possible Solutions

1. The audiologist establishes a careful protocol for testing, including a questionnaire, in order to evaluate potential benefit from amplification.
2. The audiologist decides not to provide services in the setting, as it is impossible to meet the preferred practice standards.
3. The audiologist provides a comprehensive aural rehabilitation program as follow-up to hearing aid fitting to ensure benefit from amplification.

Discussion Questions

1. Do audiologists have an obligation to develop services to fulfill unmet needs?
2. Can quality services be provided in a less than standard manner?
3. How can services be documented to demonstrate the quality of care provided?

Background Information

Alvord, L. S. (1990). Noise levels in physicians' offices. *Ear and Hearing, 11*(5), 391–393.

Schow, R. L. (1992). Hearing assessment and treatment in nursing homes. *Hearing Instruments, 43*(7), 7–11.

Schow, R. L., & Nertonne, M. A. (1977). Assessment of hearing handicap by nursing home residents and staff. *Journal of Academy of Rehabilitation Audiology, 10*, 2–12.

AUDITORY INTEGRATION TRAINING

An audiologist is treating an autistic child using "Auditory Integration Training" (AIT) developed by Guy Berard. The family was told that it is not clear who will and who will not benefit from treatment, but does not know that the procedure is considered experimental. The audiologist reported anecdotal information to the family regarding claimed successful treatment of similar children and implied that they should see comparable benefits.

Areas of ASHA's Code of Ethics That May Apply

Principle of Ethics I, Rules D and F
Principle of Ethics III, Rules C and D

Areas of AAA's Code of Ethics That May Apply

Principle 5, Rule 5a
Principle 5, Rule 5b

Possible Solutions

1. Explain the experimental status of AIT and reduce costs for enrollees.
2. Discontinue provision of AIT until research efficacy is established.
3. Develop informed consent form for parents to sign.

Discussion Questions

1. Is the treatment of autism in the scope of practice of audiologists?
2. Does a professional have an obligation to withhold treatment until efficacy is proven, even when case reports are promising?
3. Is it unethical to provide a "benign" treatment if it is unproven?
4. Should a practitioner devise a research protocol and follow it carefully with informed consent if he or she wishes to use an unproven procedure?
5. Should fees be reduced for persons participating in research when being a study subject is a condition of enrollment?
6. Does the use of case reports lead to treatment outcome expectations?

Background Information

American Speech-Language-Hearing Association. (1994). Auditory integration training. *Asha, 36*(11), 55–58.

American Academy of Audiology. (1993). Position statement—Auditory integration training. *Audiology Today, 5*(4), 21.

Friel-Patti, S. (1994). Commitment to theory. *American Journal of Speech-Language Pathology, 3*(2), 30–34.

Gravel, J. S. (1994). Auditory integration training: Placing the burden of proof. *American Journal of Speech-Language Pathology, 3*(2), 25–29.

Monville, D. K., & Nelson, N. W. (1994). Parental viewpoints on change following auditory integration training for autism. *American Journal of Speech-Language Pathology, 3*(2), 41–53.

Palm, D. E. (1994). Letters to the editor—FDA and AIT. *Audiology Today, 6* (3), 8.

Rimland, B., & Edelson, S. M. (1994). The effects of auditory integration training on autism. *American Journal of Speech-Language Pathology, 3*(2), 16–24.

Rimland, B., & Edelson, S. M. (1995). A pilot study on auditory integration training in autism. *Journal of Autism and Developmental Disorders, 25*(1), 61–70.

Veale, T. K. (1994). Auditory integration training: The use of a new listening treatment within our profession. *American Journal of Speech-Language Pathology, 3*(2), 12–15.

BILLING IMPROPRIETIES

A speech-language pathologist pads a client's attendance records and bills the insurance company for time in which the client was not seen. You are aware that your colleague is placing your agency in ethical/financial jeopardy by engaging in this practice.

Areas of ASHA's Code of Ethics That May Apply

Principle of Ethics I, Rule J
Principle of Ethics IV, Rules B and G

Possible Solutions

1. Turn the colleague in to the director of clinical services.
2. Tell the colleague that you are aware of the practice and will reveal the problem to administrator(s), if the practice is not ceased immediately.
3. Do and say nothing and hope for the best.
4. Tell another colleague in the hope that he or she will turn the person in for deceptive record keeping.
5. Request a transfer to another department.
6. Inform ASHA's Ethical Practice Board.

Discussion Questions

1. How can false claims for services be documented?
2. What are the possible consequences of failing to report this behavior?
3. What are the potential ethical and legal ramifications?

Background Information

American Speech-Language-Hearing Association. (1994). Representation of services for insurance reimbursement or funding. *Asha, 36*(Suppl. 13), 9–10.
Petersdorf, R.G. (1989). A matter of integrity. *Academic Medicine, 64*(3), 119–123.

BURNOUT AND ALCOHOLISM

An audiologist employed at a state hospital was emotionally exhausted and frequently drank excessively after work hours. She had been convicted twice for drunk driving. Occasionally in the afternoon, this audiologist drank alcohol in her office, making it necessary for another staff audiologist to cover her appointments. There have been several instances in which this audiologist has reported inaccurate test results.

Areas of ASHA's Code of Ethics That May Apply

Principle of Ethics I, Rule L

Areas of AAA's Code of Ethics That May Apply

Principle 2, Rule 2b

Possible Solutions

1. The audiologist seeks professional assistance for substance abuse.
2. The audiologist withdraws from affected areas of practice.
3. You inform the audiologist about the consequences of substance abuse on state property.

Discussion Questions

1. How can professional services be adversely affected by substance abuse?
2. How can professionals cope with colleagues who have problems related to substance abuse?
3. Have you had experience with a professional colleague with substance abuse problems? If so, how did you deal with this person?
4. If you sensed that you were struggling with substance abuse, what would you do to manage it?
5. What are the legal and ethical ramifications of failing to report a colleague who is performing clinical services while clearly under the influence of alcohol?

Background Information

Miller, M. M., & Potter, R. E. (1982). Professional burnout among speech-language pathologists. *Asha, 22*(3), 177–181.

Potter, R. E., & Rudensey, K. (1984). Coping with burnout. *Asha, 24*(11), 35–37.

Strike, K. A., & Soltis, J. F. (1992). *The ethics of teaching.* New York: Teachers College Press.

CERUMEN MANAGEMENT

An audiologist becomes frustrated over losing clients who are potential hearing aid users to otologists when she refers for cerumen removal prior to making an earmold impression. She decides to begin removing cerumen herself, even though she has had no specific training for cerumen removal.

Areas of ASHA's Code of Ethics That May Apply

Principle of Ethics II, Rule B

Areas of AAA's Code of Ethics That May Apply

Principle 2, Rule 2b

Possible Solutions

1. Attend a cerumen management training course.
2. Arrange for training with a local physician.
3. Continue the practice, being as careful as possible.

Discussion Questions

1. Is an audiologist's training program sufficient to prepare for adequate cerumen removal?
2. Is an audiologist better prepared to remove cerumen than the nurse in a doctor's office?
3. Are there any complications of cerumen removal that can create difficulty for the client?
4. Does an audiologist's liability insurance cover cerumen removal?

Background Information

Ballachanda, B. B., & Peers, C. J. (1992). Cerumen management: Instruments and procedures. *Asha, 34*(2), 43–46.
Roeser, R. J., & Crandell, C. (1991). The audiologist's responsibility in cerumen management. *Asha, 33*(1), 51–53.
Manning, R. (1992). *Cerumen management.* Lexington, KY: Robert D. Manning.

CHILD ABUSE BY AN AUDIOLOGIST

An audiologist who treats children in a private practice is convicted of child abuse in a nonwork setting.

Areas of ASHA's Code of Ethics That May Apply

Principle of Ethics I, Rule L
Principle of Ethics IV, Rule B

Areas of AAA's Code of Ethics That May Apply

Principle 1
Principle 4, Rule 4a
Principle 8, Rule 8b

Possible Solutions

1. Overlook the situation.
2. Require that the audiologist limit practice to adults.
3. Insist that clients be informed of the conviction.
4. Remove the audiologist's credentials to practice, such as CCCs, state license.

Discussion Questions

1. Is behavior that occurs "off-duty" relevant to the performance of professional duties?
2. Can behavior that has not yet caused harm in the workplace do so in the future?
3. Should conduct be sanctioned that demeans the profession in the public mind?

Background Information

Resnick, D. M. (1991). Issues in ethics: Jurisdiction, diversity and some rules of the game. *Audiology Today, 3*(6), 12–13.

COLLABORATIVE SERVICE

You have two kindergarten-age children on your caseload who are identified as language delayed and have been receiving services in a noncategorical preschool special education program. According to Bulletin 1508 of the Louisiana Department of Education (1993), "non-categorical preschool is an exceptionality in which children ages three through five, but not enrolled in a State approved kindergarten, are identified as having a condition which is described according to functional and/or developmental levels as mild/moderate or severe/profound" (p. 59). This year, these children are being mainstreamed in the mornings into a kindergarten classroom. You have been providing consultations to the special education teacher once a week and in-the-class collaborative service twice a week. You now wish to switch such an approach to the regular kindergarten setting to ensure the children's social and academic success communicatively. The teacher is enthusiastic, saying such an approach can also benefit other students in the class who are weak in language. Also, the teacher would consider the approach helpful to personal professional development. The coordinator is reluctant, saying special education should not be brought into a room for children with language differences, not deficits.

Areas of ASHA's Code of Ethics That May Apply.

Principle of Ethics III, Rules D and E
Principle of Ethics IV, Rule F

Possible Solutions

1. The Early Childhood Special Education Coordinator, teacher and SLP meet together to discuss the legal aspects of the students' entitlement to "appropriate services". . ."in the least restrictive environment" (Public Law 94-142), as well as how the benefits to the kindergarten teacher and children are outweighed by any negative aspects.
2. Articles about collaboration and its benefits, as well as the role of SLPs in sociolinguistic education, are shared with the coordinator.
3. A clearly developed, nonintrusive collaborative plan is developed by both teachers and the SLP and is presented and explained to the coordinator.

Discussion Questions

1. Are the legal aspects more compelling in this situation than the professional relationships? What are the relevant federal laws and what do they require?
2. Do state regulations conflict with these laws?

Background Information

American Speech-Language-Hearing Association. (1991). A model for collaborative service delivery for students with language-learning disorders in the public schools. *Asha, 33*(Suppl. 5), 44–50.

Beckoff, A. G., & Bender, W. N. (1989). Programming for mainstream kindergarten success in preschool: Teachers' perceptions of necessary prerequisite skills. *Journal of Early Intervention, 13,* 269–280.

Ellis, L., Schlaudecker, C., & Regimbal, C. (1995). Effectiveness of a collaborative approach to basic concept instruction with kindergarten children. *Language, Speech and Hearing Services in Schools, 26*(1), 69–74.

Louisiana Department of Education. (1993). *Pupil appraisal handbook: Bulletin 1508.* Baton Rouge: Louisiana Department of Education.

Marvin, C. (1990). Problems in school-based language consultation and collaborative services: Defining the terms and improving the process. In W. A. Secord (Ed.), *Best practices in school speech-language pathology* (pp. 37–49). San Antonio, TX: The Psychological Corporation.

Montgomery, J. K. (1992). Implementing collaborative consultation perspectives from the field: Language, speech and hearing services in schools. *Language, Speech, and Hearing Services in Schools, 23*(4), 363–364.

Nelson, N. W. (1990). Only relevant practices can be best. In W. A. Secord (Ed.), *Best practices in school speech-language pathology* (pp. 15–27). San Antonio, TX: The Psychological Corporation.

Russell, S. C., & Kaderavak, J. N. (1993). Alternative models for collaboration. *Language, Speech, and Hearing Services in Schools, 24*(2), 75–78.

Shonkoff, J. P., & Meisels, S. J. (1991). Defining eligibility for services under PL 99-457. *Journal of Early Intervention, 15,* 21–25.

Wolery, M., Venn, M. L., Schroeder, C., Holcombe, A., Huffman, K., Martin, C. G., Brookfield, J., & Fleming, L. A. (1994). A survey of the extent to which SLPs are employed in preschool programs. *Language, Speech, and Hearing Services in Schools, 24*(2), 76–78.

Wolfram, W. (1993). Research to practice: A proactive role for speech-language pathologists in sociolinguistic education. *Language, Speech, and Hearing Services in Schools, 24*(3), 181–185.

Based on material from: "Ethical considerations in the practice of speech language pathology" by B. N. Witt, 1994 November, Presentation at the meeting of the American Speech-Language-Hearing Association, New Orleans.

CONFIDENTIALITY AND TELEPHONE MESSAGE

An audiologist calls a client's office and leaves a message that Mr. Smith's hearing aid is ready to be picked up after repair.

Areas of ASHA's Code of Ethics That May Apply

Principle of Ethics I, Rule I

Areas of AAA's Code of Ethics That May Apply

Principle 3, Rule 3a

Possible Solutions

1. Leave a message with the secretary requesting a return call.
2. Send a personal note to the client.
3. Ask if personal messages are to be left with office staff.

Discussion Questions

1. Is this a violation of confidentiality?
2. Are there circumstances in which this could be acceptable?

Background Information

Rowland, R. (1986). Legal implications of a professional dispensing practice. *Seminars in Hearing, 7*(2), 193–198.
Helmick, J. W. (1994). Ethics and the profession of audiology. *Seminars in Hearing, 15*(3), 190–198.

CONTINUING EDUCATION

One practices as a speech-language pathologist, but does not read professional journals, attend continuing education activities, or make any other effort to remain current in the field.

Areas of ASHA's Code of Ethics That May Apply

Principle of Ethics II, Rule C

Possible Solutions

1. Mandatory continuing education.
2. Peer support, such as a journal club.
3. Employer provides opportunities for and ensures that speech-language pathologists continue their professional education.
4. Reward for continuing education activities.

Discussion Questions

1. What professional activities can be considered continuing education?
2. Why is continuing education important?
3. Should continuing education be mandatory or voluntary? Justify your answer.
4. Which states require continuing education for license renewal?
5. How has the practice of speech-language pathology changed in the past 5 to 10 years?
6. Should ASHA require continuing education to renew CCCs?

Background Information

Bytnar, B., & Ralph, K. (1994). The transition from student to professional. *Asha, 36*(6), 42–43.

Manning, P. R., & DeBakey, L. (1992). Lifelong learning tailored to individual clinical practice. *Journal of the American Medical Association, 268*(9), 1135–1136.

Oxman, A. D., Sackett, D. L., & Guyatt, G. H. (1993). Users' guides to the medical literature I: How to get started. *Journal of the American Medical Association, 270*(17), 2093–2095.

DEMARKETING

A speech-language pathologist makes fewer recommendations for needed speech-language treatment to have more time available to provide speech-language evaluations. The fee for speech-language evaluations is considerably higher than for treatment.

Areas of ASHA's Code of Ethics That May Apply

Principle of Ethics I, Rule A
Principle of Ethics III, Rule B

Possible Solutions

1. Audit the clinical services.
2. Revise the fee schedule, so that diagnostic and treatment services are commensurate.
3. Notify the speech-language pathologist of the inappropriateness of this practice.
4. Review ASHA's statements about conflicts of professional interest.
5. Discuss the responsibility of SLPs to hold paramount the welfare of their consumers.

Discussion Questions

1. What circumstances can create the appearance of demarketing treatment services?
2. How can the potential for demarketing of treatment services be avoided?

Background Information

American Speech-Language-Hearing Association. (1994). Conflicts of professional interest. *Asha, 36*(Suppl. 13), 7–8.

DYSPHAGIA TRAINING

A speech-language pathologist (SLP) is not trained to provide treatment for dysphagia, but has been assigned five clients with swallowing disorders. No continuing education and no funds or time off are available for such training. The SLP expresses concerns to the program director. The program director, also a speech-language pathologist, advises the SLP to "wing it" until there are funds for a dysphagia training program.

Areas of ASHA's Code of Ethics That May Apply

Principle of Ethics I, Rule A
Principle of Ethics II, Rules B and E

Possible Solutions

1. Inform the program director that both of you are violating the ASHA Code of Ethics as well as the code of ethics of the state association

and licensure board and are subject to sanctions, including loss of certification and/or licensure.

2. Locate local resources.

Discussion Questions

1. What are the potential risks to dysphagia clients?
2. How could the speech-language pathologist gain the necessary skills to meet these clients' needs?
3. Could incompetent provision of services harm these clients?

Background Information

American Speech-Language-Hearing Association. (1990). Knowledge and skills needed by speech-language pathologists providing services to dysphagic patients-clients. *Asha, 32*(Suppl. 2), 7–12.

Groher, M. E. (1992). *Dysphagia: Diagnosis and management.* Boston: Butterworth-Heinemann.

DYSPHAGIA TREATMENT

In treating a client for dysphagia, feeding is initiated too early which leads to choking and aspiration pneumonia.

Areas of ASHA's Code of Ethics That May Apply

Principle of Ethics I, Rule A
Principle of Ethics II, Rule B

Possible Solutions

1. Review evaluation and treatment criteria for dysphagia.
2. Consult with and observe other speech-language pathologists treating clients with dysphagia.
3. Obtain written orders from the attending physician for evaluation and treatment of dysphagia.

Discussion Questions

1. How should the need for dysphagia services be determined?
2. Can incompetent provision of services harm the client?
3. How much and what type of training is needed to provide competent services to dysphagia clients?
4. Does it matter if a physician's written orders to initiate feeding were on the chart?

Background Information

American Speech-Language-Hearing Association. (1994). The protection of rights of people receiving audiology or speech-language pathology services. *Asha, 36*(1), 60–63.

Arvedson, J. C., & Brudsky, L. (1993). *Pediatric swallowing and feeding: Assessment and management*. San Diego: Singular Publishing Group.

Kasprisin, A. T., Clumeck, N., & Niro-Murcia, M. (1989). The efficacy of rehabilitation management of dysphagia. *Dysphagia, 4*, 48–52.

Logemann, J. A. (1983). *Evaluation and treatment of swallowing disorders*. San Diego: College-Hill Press.

Logemann, J. A. (1986). Treatment for aspiration related to dysphagia: An overview. *Dysphagia, 1*, 34–38.

Lynch, C. (1986). Harm to the public: Is it real? *Asha, 28*(6), 25–31.

Martin, B. J. W., Corlew, M., Wood, H., Olson, D., Golopol, L., Wingo, M., & Kirmani, N. (1994). The association of swallowing dysfunction and aspiration pneumonia. *Dysphagia, 9*, 1–6.

Thomasma, D. C. (1992–1993). The ethics of caring for vulnerable individuals. *National Student Speech-Language-Hearing Association Journal, 20*, 122–124.

ELECTRONIC BREACH OF CONFIDENTIALITY

Your hospital setting uses an electronic network to store patient information. A hospital supplies company is contacting families of patients seen at your hospital in an effort to sell various products. According to family members, the representative appears to have information about each patient's condition. You suspect a breach of electronic security.

Areas of ASHA's Code of Ethics That May Apply

Principle of Ethics I, Rule I

Areas of AAA's Code of Ethics That May Apply

Principle 3, Rule 3a

Possible Solutions

1. Report the problem to the hospital administrator.
2. Contact the department that oversees the electronic system used to manage client data.

Discussion Questions

1. Who is responsible for maintaining confidentiality of electronic records?
2. Are the problems associated with an electronic database greater than the advantages?
3. Is it possible to maintain confidentiality of electronic records? What are some safeguards?
4. Is the hospital at fault? Should hospital legal representatives be notified and consulted? Explain.

Background Information

Darr, K. (1991). *Ethics in health services management.* Baltimore: Health Professions Press.

Flower, R. M. (1984). *Delivery of speech-language pathology and audiology services.* Baltimore: Williams and Wilkins.

Garrett, T. M., Baillie, H. W., & Garrett, R. M. (1989). *Health care ethics.* Englewood Cliffs, NJ: Prentice Hall.

Silverman, F. H. (1992). *Legal-ethical considerations, restrictions, and obligations for clinicians who treat communicative disorders.* Springfield, IL: Charles D. Thomas.

EXPIRATION OF FINANCIAL BENEFITS

An audiologist is seeing a client for aural rehabilitation services. His insurance plan will pay for four visits. At the end of four visits, progress has been made in adjustment to amplification, speech-reading skills, and coping strategy development; however, it does not appear that this client has achieved his maximum function.

Areas of ASHA's Code of Ethics That May Apply

Principle of Ethics I

Areas of AAA's Code of Ethics That May Apply

Principle 1, Rule 1a

Possible Solutions

1. During the four visits that were covered, the audiologist could have included the family or a significant other. It is possible to extend services through appropriate sharing of responsibilities.
2. The audiologist can continue to see the client without compensation.
3. The audiologist can continue to see the client, but the client will have to cover services beyond the limit of his insurance plan.
4. The audiologist can discontinue seeing the client when the insurance benefit runs out.
5. The audiologist may be able to arrange group therapy for the client at a lower price and seek an agreement from the insurance company to cover more visits.

Discussion Questions

1. Does an audiologist ethically have to continue services, if it means a financial loss?
2. Can employers pressure professionals to cease services when insurance money runs out?
3. Will quality of services decline if support personnel or family are involved?
4. When can group therapy be justified?

Background Information

American Medical Association, Council on Ethical and Judicial Affairs. (1995). Ethical issues in managed care. *Journal of the American Medical Association, 273*(4), 330–335.

American Speech-Language-Hearing Association. (1995). *Managing managed care: A practical guide for audiologists and speech-language pathologists.* Rockville, MD: Author.

FABRICATING EVALUATION RESULTS

A speech-language pathologist writes a speech-language evaluation report on a client who was observed and tested by a speech-language pathologist who suddenly resigned and left the area without writing a report or filing the test results.

Areas of ASHA's Code of Ethics That May Apply

Principle of Ethics I, Rules A, H, and J
Principle of Ethics IV, Rules B and C

Possible Solutions

1. Reschedule the speech-language evaluation and charge for only one assessment.
2. Refer the client to another speech-language pathologist.
3. Review the ASHA Code of Ethics.
4. Develop a documentation system for record keeping and reporting.
5. Inform the absent speech-language pathologist's supervisor of the problem and possible consequence.

Discussion Questions

1. How could it be determined that the report was completed by a speech-language pathologist who never observed or tested the client?
2. Is the speech-language pathologist falsifying evaluation information to obtain funding?
3. Was information falsified to keep the program in compliance with accreditation standards?

Background Information

American Speech-Language-Hearing Association. (1994). Representation of services for insurance reimbursement or funding. *Asha, 36*(Suppl. 13), 9–10.
American Speech-Language-Hearing Association. (1994). *Professional Services Board standards and accreditation manual.* Rockville, MD: Author.
American Speech-Language-Hearing Association. (1994). Professional liability and risk management for the audiology and speech-language pathology profession. *Asha, 36*(Suppl. 12), 25–38.

FACILITATED COMMUNICATION

You are a speech-language pathologist at a residential facility for children with autism. Several of the parents and staff members strongly suggest that you develop a program involving implementation of facilitated communication.

Areas of ASHA's Code of Ethics That May Apply

Principle of Ethics I, Rule E

Possible Solutions

1. Develop and implement a program of facilitated communication.
2. Explain ASHA's position on facilitated communication.
3. Refer to another speech-language pathologist.
4. Do a literature search on facilitated communication and set up a research project involving field testing of the program with selected children within the facility.

Discussion Questions

1. What evidence is available to support facilitated communication?
2. What are the possible negative consequences of facilitated communication?
3. What is ASHA's position on facilitated communication?
4. What concerns need to be addressed about methods for augmenting communication skills of persons with communication disabilities?

Background Information

American Speech-Language-Hearing Association. (1994). Urgent: Response needed for facilitated communication. *Asha, 36*(11), 7.

American Speech-language-Hearing Association. (1995, March). Position statement: Facilitated communication. *Asha, 37*(Suppl. 14), 22.

Biklen, D. (1992). Typing to talk: Facilitated communication. *American Journal of Speech-Language Pathology, 1*(2), 15–17.

Biklen, D. (1992). Facilitated communication: Biklen responds. *American Journal of Speech-Language Pathology, 1*(2), 21–22.

Calculator, S. N. (1992). Perhaps the emperor has clothes after all: A response to Biklen. *American Journal of Speech-Language Pathology, 1*(2), 18–20.

Calculator, S. N. (1992). Facilitated communication: Calculator responds. *American Journal of Speech-Language Pathology, 1*(2), 23–24.

Calculator, S. N., & Hatch, E. R. (1995). Validation of facilitated communication: A case study and beyond. *American Journal of Speech-Language Pathology, 4*(1), 49–58.

Crossley, R. (1992). Lending a hand: A personal account of the development of facilitated communication training. *American Journal of Speech-Language Pathology, 1*(3), 15–18.

McLean, J. (1992). Facilitated communication: Some thoughts on Biklen's and Calculator's interaction. *American Journal of Speech-Language Pathology, 1*(2), 25–27.

Shane, H. C., & Kearns, K. (1994). An examination of the role of the facilitator in "Facilitated Communication." *American Journal of Speech-Language Pathology, 3*(3), 48–54.

FAILURE TO REFER

A speech-language pathologist disregards a 48-year-old man's complaint of pain and hoarseness. He was referred for trial voice therapy. Five years earlier, the man was seen by an otolaryngologist who reported the presence of a normal-appearing larynx.

Areas of ASHA's Code of Ethics That May Apply

Principle of Ethics I, Rules A and B

Possible Solutions

1. Provision of continuing professional education.
2. Refer to a speech-language pathologist knowledgeable about diagnosis and treatment of voice disorders.
3. Refer directly to an otolaryngologist.

Discussion Questions

1. Would it matter when the pain and hoarseness began?
2. Would sudden or gradual onset matter?
3. Would it matter if the problems were accompanied by swallowing difficulties or nasal regurgitation of solids or fluids?

4. What would be best practice if there were periods of no pain or hoarseness?
5. What might be the outcome of delaying medical referral?

Background Information

Aronson, A. E. (1990). *Clinical voice disorders.* New York: Thieme, Inc.
Case, J. L. (1991). *Clinical management of voice disorders.* Austin, TX: PRO-ED.
Lynch, C. (1986). Harm to the public: Is it real? *Asha, 28*(6), 25–31.

FALSIFYING CREDENTIALS

A clinical fellow in speech-language pathology falsified an ASHA membership card and a Certificate of Clinical Competence in an effort to appear to clients as being a fully credentialed speech-language pathologist.

Areas of ASHA's Code of Ethics That May Apply

Principle of Ethics III, Rule A
Principle of Ethics IV, Rules A and B

Possible Solutions

1. Inform the clinical fellow about professional repercussions for falsifying credentials and deceiving consumers.
2. Inform the clinical fellow's supervisor about the problem.
3. The clinical fellow's supervisor refuses to continue supervising the individual.
4. Inform ASHA's Committee on Certification.
5. Inform ASHA's Ethical Practice Board.

Discussion Questions

1. What may have caused the clinical fellow to falsify professional credentials?
2. Would it matter if the clinical fellowship supervisor was aware of the ethical violation?
3. Is it the responsibility of the clinical fellowship supervisor to review the Codes of Ethical Practice with clinical fellows?

4. Was the quality of clinical services compromised by the clinical fellow's behavior?

Background Information

American Speech-Language-Hearing Association. (1994). Clinical fellowship supervisor's responsibilities. *Asha, 36*(Suppl. 13), 22–23.

FALSIFYING RECORDS

The Heathcliff and Garfield Corporation hires speech-language pathologists to provide contracted services to nursing home residents. The speech-language pathologists are instructed to provide the maximum services allowed to residents with Medicare benefits and to document progress, even if a client does not respond or make progress toward meeting objectives.

Areas of ASHA's Code of Ethics That May Apply

Principle of Ethics I, Rules E, H, and J
Principle of Ethics III, Rule C
Principle of Ethics IV, Rules B and E

Possible Solutions

1. Inform the area corporation supervisor that the practice is out of compliance with professional ethics.
2. Inform ASHA's Ethical Practice Board.
3. Consult with other speech-language pathologists providing contract services.

Discussion Questions

1. If the speech-language pathologist engages in the practices advocated by the corporation, who is legally and ethically responsible?
2. Are the credentials of the speech-language pathologists working for the corporation at-risk?
3. What motivates such practices?

4. Should other area speech-language pathologists become involved in this matter? Why? How?

Background Information

American Speech-Language-Hearing Association. (1994). Representation of services for insurance reimbursement or funding. *Asha, 36*(Suppl. 13), 9–10.

FINANCIAL CONFLICT OF INTEREST: STOCK OWNERSHIP

An audiologist buys stock in a company that manufactures hearing aids and he continues to recommend and sell that company's products.

Areas of ASHA's Code of Ethics That May Apply

Principle of Ethics III, Rules B, C, and E

Areas of AAA's Code of Ethics That May Apply

Principle 4, Rule 4c
Principle 5, Rules 5a and 5b

Possible Solutions

1. Keep the stock and continue dispensing hearing aids.
2. Sell the stock and continue dispensing hearing aids.
3. Quit dispensing hearing aids made by that company.
4. Inform clients of possible bias.

Discussion Questions

1. Does a professional have a right to benefit financially from personal information about companies?
2. Does the number of hearing aids one audiologist can sell actually affect the "bottom line" of a manufacturer?

3. Is the appearance of conflict of interest as important as an actual conflict of interest?

Background Information

American Speech-Language-Hearing Association. (1994). Conflicts of professional interest. *Asha, 36*(Suppl. 13), 7–8.

Curran, J., & Harford, E. (1991). Point: Counterpoint. *Audiology Today, 3*(6), 14–16.

Friel-Patti, S. (1994). Professional ethics and the marketplace. *Texas Speech-Language-Hearing Association Communicologist, 19*(6), 5–6.

Resnick, D. M. (1991). Issues in ethics: An introduction to ethics. *Audiology Today, 3*(5), 13–14.

Resnick, D. M. (1992). Issues in ethics: Balancing the ethics of a profession and a business. *Audiology Today, 4*(2), 18–20.

Resnick, D. M. (1992). Issues in ethics: Ethics and good friends are similar. *Audiology Today, 4*(3), 12–13.

GUARANTEED RESULTS

An audiologist circulates literature claiming to be the only person capable of administering a self-developed method promised to be the only cure for tinnitus.

Areas of ASHA's Code of Ethics That May Apply

Principle of Ethics I, Rules D and F
Principle of Ethics III

Areas of AAA's Code of Ethics That May Apply

Principle 5, Rules 5a and 5b
Principle 6, Rule 6b

Possible Solutions

1. Inform the audiologist that these practices are unethical and will not be tolerated by the professional community.

2. File a complaint with ASHA's Ethical Practice Board and the state's licensing board.

Discussion Questions

1. Does it matter where the literature has been circulated?
2. Does it matter what consumers report about the outcome of the method?
3. Would it matter if the audiologist was aware that this practice is unethical?
4. How would area ENT physicians be aware of the audiologist's claims?
5. What actions might ENT physicians take?

Background Information

Kodama, A., Kitahara, M., & Komada, K. (1994). Tinnitus evaluation using the tinnitus grading system. *Acta Otolaryngology, 510*(Suppl.), 62–66.

Matsuhira, T., Yamashita, K., & Yasuda, M. (1992). Estimation of the loudness of tinnitus from matching tests. *British Journal of Audiology, 26*(6), 387–395.

Mitchell, C. R., Vernon, J. A., & Creedon, T. A. (1993). Measuring tinnitus parameters: Loudness, pitch, and maskability. *Journal American Academy Audiology, 4*(3), 139–151.

Moller, A. R., Moller, M. B., Jannetta, P. J., & Jho, H. D. (1992). Compound action potentials recorded from the exposed eighth nerve in patients with intractable tinnitus. *Laryngoscope, 102*(2), 187–197.

Newman, C. W., Wharton, J. A., Shivapuja, B. G., & Jacobson, G. P. (1994). Relationships among psychoacoustic judgments, speech understanding ability and self-perceived handicap in tinnitus subjects. *Audiology, 33*(1), 47–60.

Okusa, M., Shiraishi, T., Kubo, T., & Matsunaga, T. (1993). Tinnitus suppression by electrical promontory stimulation in sensorineural deaf patients. *Acta Otolaryngology, 501*(Suppl.), 54–58.

Phoon, W. H., Lee, H. S., & Chia, S. E. (1993). Tinnitus in noise-exposed workers. *Occupational Medicine, 43*(1), 35–38.

Shemesh, Z., Attias, J., Ornan, N., Shapira, N., & Shahar, A. (1993). Vitamin B12 deficiency in patients with chronic-tinnitus and noise-induced hearing loss. *American Journal of Otolaryngology, 14*(2), 94–99.

Shupak, A., Bar-El, E., Podoshin, L., Spitzer, O., Gordon, C. R., & Ben-David, J. (1994). Vestibular findings associated with chronic noise induced hearing impairment. *Acta Otolaryngology, 114*(6), 579–585.

Vernon, J., Griest, S., & Press, L. (1992). Attributes of tinnitus that may predict tempore mandibular joint dysfunction. *Cranio, 10*(4), 282–287, 287–288.

HEARING SCREENING

A speech-language pathologist who is employed by a hospital rehabilitation program is told that hearing screening is not necessary for patients in the program.

Areas of ASHA's Code of Ethics That May Apply

Principle of Ethics I, Rules A and B

Possible Solutions

1. Provide the supervisor with appropriate information from the Code of Ethics and ASHA's Preferred Practice Patterns.
2. Ignore the situation.
3. Refer patients for hearing evaluation by an audiologist.
4. Initiate appropriate paper-and-pencil screening procedures for patients seen personally.
5. Report the situation to state and national regulatory bodies.

Discussion Questions

1. What if you ignore the situation and it is reported by someone else?
2. What if patients follow the recommendation for hearing evaluation?
3. What if you ignore the situation and later learn that a patient's lack of progress has been from a hearing impairment?
4. What if the supervisor disregards the information provided?

Background Information

American Speech-Language-Hearing Association. (1992). Considerations in screening adults/older persons for handicapping hearing impairments. *Asha, 34*(9), 81–87.

American Speech-Language-Hearing Association. (1993). Preferred practice patterns. *Asha*(Suppl. 11), 5.

Coren, S., & Kakstian, A. R. (1992). The development and cross-validation of a self-report inventory to assess pure-tone threshold hearing sensitivity. *Journal of Speech and Hearing Research, 35*, 921–928.

Frank, T., & Petersen, D. R. (1987). Accuracy of a 40 dB HL audioscope and audiometer screening for adults. *Ear and Hearing, 8*(3), 180–193.

Lichtenstein, J. J., Bess, F. H., & Logan, S. A. (1988). Validation of screening tools for identifying hearing-impaired elderly in primary care. *Journal of the American Medical Association, 259*(19), 2875–2878.

McBride, W. S., Mulrow, C. D., Aguilar, C., & Tuley, M. R. (1994). Methods for screening for hearing loss in older adults. *American Journal of the Medical Sciences, 307*(1), 40–42.

Newman, C. W., Weinstein, B. E., Jacobson, G. P., & Hug, C. A. (1990). The hearing handicap inventory for adults: Psychometric adequacy and audiometric correlates. *Ear and Hearing, 11*(6), 430–433.

Ventry, I. M., & Weinstein, B. E. (1983). Identification of elderly people with hearing problems. *Asha, 25*(7), 37–42.

HIV ISSUES—1

A speech-language pathologist refuses to treat a client who is HIV positive.

Areas of ASHA's Code of Ethics That May Apply

Principle of Ethics I, Rule C

Possible Solutions

1. Prevent the transmission of HIV to the highest degree possible.
2. Follow procedures for preventing disease transmission.

Discussion Questions

1. What populations and settings are at high risk for HIV?
2. What precautionary measures should be taken by speech-language pathologists and audiologists working with clients who have HIV?
3. What guidelines for infection control does your facility use?
4. What Professional Services Board standards address infection control?
5. How can compliance with universal precautions for exposure to blood and body substances from HIV positive patients be encouraged?

Background Information

American Speech-Language-Hearing Association. (1989). AIDS/HIV: Report: Implications for speech-language pathologists and audiologists. *Asha, 29,* 33–37.

American Speech-Language-Hearing Association. (1990). AIDS/HIV: Implications for speech-language pathologists and audiologists. *Asha, 30*, 46–48.

American Speech-Language-Hearing Association. (1994). *Professional Services Board standards and accreditation manual.* Rockville, MD: Author.

Darr, K. (1991). *Ethics in health sciences management.* Baltimore: Health Professions Press.

Flower, W. M., & Sooty, C. D. (1987). AIDS: An introduction for speech-language pathologists and audiologists. *Asha, 27*(11), 25–30.

Grube, M. M., & Nunley, R. L. (1995). Current infection control practices in speech-language pathology. *American Journal of Speech-Language Pathology, 4*(2), 14–23.

Kemp, R. (1994). Practicing office safety in the 90's: Infection control for audiologists. *Audiology Today, 6*(5), 23–25.

Kemp, R. J., Roeser, R. J., Pearson, D. W., & Ballchandra, B. B. (1995). *Infection control for the professions of speech-language pathology and audiology.* Chesterfield, MO: Oaktree Products, Inc.

Kulpa, J. I., Blackstone, S. W., Clarke, C. C., Collignon, M. M., Griffin, E. B., Hutchins, B. F., Jernigan, L. R., Mellott, K. E., Rao, P. R., Frattali, C. M., & Seymour, C. M. (1991). Chronic communicable diseases and risk management in the school. *Language, Speech, and Hearing Services in Schools, 22*(1), 345–352.

Lubinski, R. (1994). Infection prevention. In R. Lubinski & C. Frattali (Eds.), *Professional issues in speech-language pathology and audiology* (pp. 269–281). San Diego: Singular Publishing Group.

McMillan, M. D., & Willette, S. J. (1988). Aseptic technique: A procedure for prevention of disease transmission in the practice environment. *Asha, 30*(11), 35–37.

Pressman, H. (1992). Communication disorders and dysphagia in pediatric AIDS. *Asha, 34*(1), 45–47.

Smith, K., Brandell, M. E., Poynor, R. E., & Tetchell, R. H. (1993). Infection control procedures in universities. *Asha, 33*(6), 59–62.

Strax, T. E. (1994). Ethical issues of treating patients with AIDS in a rehabilitation setting. *Journal of Physical Medicine and Rehabilitation, 73*(4), 293–295.

Zarrella, S. (1995, March 31). Infection control in cerumen management. *ADVANCE for Speech-language Pathologists and Audiologists, 5*(10), 6.

HIV ISSUES—2

You are the clinical director in a rehabilitation hospital setting. A pregnant speech-language pathologist in your unit refuses to treat a client who is HIV positive.

Areas of ASHA's Code of Ethics That May Apply

Principle of Ethics I, Rule C

Possible Solutions

1. Provide information about HIV, along with a review of hospital policies and procedures for treating patients with communicable diseases.
2. Give the speech-language pathologist notice that termination proceedings will be initiated if she continues to refuse to provide treatment.
3. Turn the matter over to the hospital director.
4. Assign the patient to a different speech-language pathologist.

Discussion Questions

1. Would it matter if the speech-language pathologist would provide services to this client if she were not pregnant?
2. Should the threat of the cytomegalovirus (CMV) that infects many AIDS patients be considered a legitimate reason for a pregnant speech-language pathologist or audiologist to resist contact with these patients during pregnancy?

Background Information (Please refer to HIV Issues—1)

Brecker, L. R. (November 8, 1993). Ethics of HIV: Fears, rights and confidentiality. *ADVANCE for Speech-Language Pathologists and Audiologists, 3*(23), 15, 24.

INADEQUATE BILINGUAL SERVICES

A school district has a large population of bilingual students and few bilingual speech-language pathologists. There is a long waiting list of students needing testing in Spanish.

Areas of ASHA's Code of Ethics That May Apply

Principle of Ethics I, Rules A, B, and C

Possible Solutions

1. Bilingual speech-language pathologists in the district could be assigned to test all children in the district needing testing in Spanish.
2. Bilingual speech-language pathologist assistants or paraprofessionals could be assigned to monolingual speech-language pathologists in schools with large populations of bilingual students to assist with testing and therapy in Spanish under direct supervision of the ASHA-certified and state licensed speech-language pathologist.
3. Additional bilingual speech-language pathologists could be recruited to work in the district.

Discussion Questions

1. Would bilingual speech-language pathologists in the district need to be experienced and trained to test in Spanish?
2. Should bilingual speech-language pathologists be assigned to the schools with predominately monolingual students?
3. Should the school district provide continuing education on the topic of testing bilingual students?

Background Information

Campbell, L. R., Brennan, D. G., & Steckol, K. F. (1992). Preservice training to meet the needs of people from diverse cultural backgrounds. *Asha, 34*(12), 29–32.

Damico, J. S., & Damico, S. K. (1993). Language and social skills from a diversity perspective: Considerations for the speech-language pathologist. *Language, Speech and Hearing Services in Schools, 24*(4), 236–243.

Roseberry-McKibbin, D. (1994). Assessment and intervention for children with limited English proficiency and language disorders. *American Journal of Speech-Language Pathology, 3*(3), 77–88.

Schiff-Myers, N. B. (1992). Considering arrested language development and language loss in the assessment of second language learners. *Language, Speech and Hearing Services in Schools, 23*(1), 28–33.

INADEQUATE CF SUPERVISION

A speech-language pathologist accepts a Clinical Fellowship position in a private practice setting. The speech-language pathologist's request for assistance with certain clients are ignored by the Clinical Fellowship supervisor.

Areas of ASHA's Code of Ethics That May Apply

Principle of Ethics I, Rule A
Principle of Ethics II, Rule D
Principle of Ethics IV, Rule A

Possible Solutions

1. Review the requirements for the Clinical Fellowship experience with the supervisor.
2. Request another Clinical Fellowship supervisor.

Discussion Questions

1. Should ASHA's Ethical Practice Board be involved?
2. Should the Clinical Fellowship speech-language pathologist receive credit for the unsupervised Clinical Fellowship experience?
3. What qualities should a new graduate speech-language pathologist look for in a Clinical Fellowship supervisor.

Background Information

American Speech-Language-Hearing Association. (1994). Clinical fellowship supervisor's responsibility. *Asha, 36*(Suppl. 13), 22–23.

INADEQUATE RECORD KEEPING

A speech-language pathologist resigned from a school district after working for an entire year without maintaining any records. The speech-language pathologist hired to replace the speech-language pathologist is assigned to do the necessary testing and paperwork for all admissions, reviews, and dismissals for the program to be in compliance.

Areas of ASHA' Code of Ethics That May Apply

Principle of Ethics I, Rule H

Possible Solutions

1. Report the departed speech-language pathologist to the state license board and to ASHA's Ethical Practice Board.
2. Provide a speech-language pathologist with experience working in the district to assist the new speech-language pathologist with the "reconstruction" task.
3. Develop a monitoring procedure to determine compliance throughout the school year.

Discussion Questions

1. Does it matter if the outgoing speech-language pathologist was licensed by the state and certified by ASHA? If not, can the individual be penalized for unethical practice?
2. Were administrative representatives of the school district responsible for monitoring paperwork within the program?
3. Should a newly hired speech-language pathologist be assigned a caseload so much out of record-keeping compliance?
4. Who is responsible for reporting this incident?
5. Is it possible for school districts to screen applicants more carefully? How?

Background Information

American Speech-Language-Hearing Association. (1991). *Report writing in the field of communication disorders: A handbook for students and clinicians.* Rockville, MD: Author.

Middleton, G., Pannbacker, M., Vekovius, G., Sanders, K., & Puett, V. (1992). *Report writing for speech-language pathologists.* Tucson, AZ: Communication Skill Builders.

INCOMPETENCY

A speech-language pathologist in private practice sees a young boy for eight sessions. The major emphasis of these sessions is conditioning for a hearing evaluation. Thresholds are reported as 15 dB. A previous hearing evaluation was completed in one session by an audiologist.

Areas of ASHA's Code of Ethics That May Apply

Principle of Ethics I, Rules A, B, C, and E
Principle of Ethics IV, Rule B

Possible Solutions

1. Notify state licensure board and/or ASHA.
2. Discuss improprieties with the speech-language pathologist.
3. Ignore the situation.
4. Encourage professional development about hearing screening by speech-language pathologists.

Discussion Questions

1. Were an unreasonable number of treatment sessions scheduled?
2. Why might this many sessions have been conducted?
3. How do ASHA's Code of Ethics and Scope of Practice relate to this situation?

Background Information

American Speech-Language-Hearing Association. (1990). Scope of practice. *Asha, 32*(Suppl. 2), 1.
American Speech-Language-Hearing Association. (1990). Guidelines for screening for hearing impairment and middle ear disorders. *Asha, 32*(Suppl. 2), 17–24.

INDIRECT EVALUATION

Based on a speech evaluation, a certified and licensed speech-language pathologist described a child's resonance as moderately hypernasal and articulation as characterized by nasal emission accompanying production of pressure consonants. The child was recommended for evaluation by a craniofacial team. The parents contacted a friend who is a speech-language pathologist in another city. Based on a brief conversation with the child over the telephone, the consulting speech-language pathologist told the parents that the child's speech was essentially normal and that there was no evidence to support the referral to a craniofacial team.

Areas of ASHA's Code of Ethics That May Apply

Principle of Ethics I, Rule G
Principle of Ethics IV

Possible Solutions

1. Refer the parents to another local speech-language pathologist for a full second-opinion evaluation.
2. Discuss the contradictory findings with the speech-language pathologist who evaluated the child's speech on the phone.

Discussion Questions

1. Would the qualifications of the speech-language pathologist who consulted by phone determine the ethics of this situation?
2. Why might the parents have been more willing to accept findings and recommendations based on indirect rather than direct evaluation of their child's speech?

Background Information

D'Antonio, L. L., & Scherer, N. J. (1995). The evaluation of speech disorders associated with clefting. In R. J. Shprintzen & J. Bardach (Eds.), *Cleft palate speech management: A multidisciplinary approach* (pp. 176–220). St. Louis: Mosby.

McWilliams, B. J., Morris, H. L., & Shelton, R. L. (1990). *Cleft palate speech*. Philadelphia: B. C. Decker, Jr.

Morris, H. L. (1992). Some questions and answers about velopharyngeal dysfunction during speech. *American Journal of Speech-Language Pathology, 1*(2), 26–28.

Shprintzen, R. J. (1992). Assessment of velopharyngeal function: Nasopharyngoscopy and multiview video fluoroscopy. In L. Brodsky, L. Holt, & D. H. Ritter-Schmidt (Eds.), *Craniofacial anomalies: An interdisciplinary approach* (pp. 196–207). St. Louis: Mosby Year Book.

Trost-Cardamone, J. E., & Bernthal, J. E. (1993). Articulation assessment procedures and treatment decisions. In K. T. Moller & C. D. Starr (Eds.),

Cleft palate: Interdisciplinary issues and treatment (pp. 307–336). Austin, TX: PRO-ED.

Witzel, M. A. (1993). Teams and teamwork: Cleft lip and palate and craniofacial treatment. *Asha, 35*(6), 42–43.

LACK OF ADHERENCE TO UNIVERSAL PRECAUTIONS

A speech-language pathologist refuses to wash hands between clients, wear latex gloves when required and appropriate, disinfect toys and furniture after each use, and take precautions when a client is bleeding.

Areas of ASHA's Code of Ethics That May Apply

Principle of Ethics I

Possible Solutions

1. Review the universal precautions with all staff in the facility.
2. Inform the speech-language pathologist that universal precautions must be followed.

Discussion Questions

1. Why might a speech-language pathologist be careless about following universal precautions?
2. Might time constraints contribute to the problem? Is this valid?
3. Can an agency allow the practice to continue?

Background Information

Grube, M. M., & Nunley, R. L. (1995). Current infection control practices in speech-language pathology. *American Journal of Speech-Language Pathology, 4*(2), 14–23.

Hegde, M. N., & Davis, D. (1995). *Clinical methods and practicum in speech-language pathology.* San Diego: Singular Publishing Group. Health and safety precautions, pp. 75–78.

Kemp, R. J., Roeser, R. J., Pearson, D. W., & Ballachanda, B. B. (1995). *Infection control for the professions of speech-language pathology and audiology.* Chesterfield, MO: Oaktree Products, Inc.

Kulpa, J. I., Blackstone, S. W., Clarke, C. C., Collignon, M. M., Griffin, E. B., Hutchins, B. F., Jernigan, L. R., Mellott, K. E., Rao, P. R., Frattali, C. M., & Seymour, C. M. (1991). Chronic communicable diseases and risk management in the schools. *Language, Speech, and Hearing Services in Schools, 22*(1), 345–352.

Lubinski, R. (1994). Infection prevention. In R. Lubinski & C. Frattali (Eds.), *Professional issues in speech-language pathology and audiology* (pp. 269–281). San Diego: Singular Publishing Group.

McMillan, M. D., & Willette, S. J. (1988). Aseptic technique: A procedure for prevention of disease transmission in the practice environment. *Asha, 30*(11), 35–37.

LACK OF INDEPENDENT PROFESSIONAL JUDGMENT

A child has been medically diagnosed with vocal nodules. On evaluation of the child's voice, which the speech-language pathologist perceives to be hoarse, rough, and hyperfunctional, and a history that indicates regular vocal abuses, the clinician recommends voice treatment. The parents then inform the clinician that the physician must refer the child for treatment for the insurance carrier to approve voice treatment. The physician will not refer until the nodules are surgically removed. The clinician then adjusts the recommendation for voice treatment to follow any recommended medical intervention by the otolaryngologist.

Areas of ASHA's Code of Ethics That May Apply

Principle of Ethics I
Principle of Ethics IV, Rule E

Possible Solutions

1. Call the physician to discuss management options.
2. Indicate to the parents the benefits that reduction of vocal abuses may have on the vocal mechanism.
3. Parents discuss options with the surgeon.
4. Parents arrange to pay for the services without reimbursement.
5. Retain a quality audiotaped voice sample.

Discussion Questions

1. What does the research indicate about the results of early surgery versus clinical management on juvenile vocal nodules?

2. Is reimbursement a viable reason for compromising independent professional judgment?

Background Information

Allen, M. S., Pettit, J. M., & Sherblom, J. D. (1991). Management of vocal nodules: A regional survey of otolaryngologists and speech-language pathologists. *Journal of Speech and Hearing Research, 34*(2), 229–235.

Colton, R. H., & Casper, J. K. (1990). *Understanding voice problems.* Baltimore: Williams & Wilkins. Chapter 4, Voice misuse and abuse: Effects on laryngeal physiology, (pp. 73–106).

Dobres, R., Lee, L., Stemple, J. C., Kummer, A. W., & Kretschmer, L. W. (1990). Description of laryngeal pathologies in children evaluated by otolaryngologists. *Journal of Speech and Hearing Disorders, 55*, 526–532.

Lancer, J. M., Syder, D., Jones, A. S., & LeBoutillieu, A. (1988). Vocal cord nodules: A review. *Clinics of Otolaryngology, 13*(1), 43–51.

McFarlane, S. C., & Watterson, T. L. (1990). Vocal nodules: Endoscopic study of their variations and treatment. *Seminars in Speech and Language, 11*(1), 47–59.

Moran, M. J., & Pentz, A. L. (1987). Otolaryngologists' opinions of voice therapy for vocal nodules in children. *Language, Speech, and Hearing Services in Schools, 18*, 172–178.

Sataloff, R. T., Speigal, J. R., & Rosen, D. C. (1993). Vocal fold scar and vocal fold nodules. *Ear, Nose and Throat Journal, 72*(8), 517.

Verdolini-Marston, K., Burke, M. K., Lessac, A., Glaze, L., & Caldwell, E. (1995). Preliminary study of two methods of treatment for laryngeal nodules. *Journal of Voice, 9*(1), 74–85.

MEDICAID

There are few ASHA-certified speech-language pathologists working in an area public school system. These clinicians have been instructed to sign Medicaid claim forms for children they do not know and to whom they have never provided services.

Areas of ASHA's Code of Ethics That May Apply

Principle of Ethics I, Rules G and J
Principle of Ethics III, Rule C

Possible Solutions

1. Work with the district to effect change in billing third-party payers.
2. Meet with the district as a group to explain concern about being asked to violate ASHA's Code of Ethics along with the possible legal ramifications.
3. Consult the state professional association, state licensure board, and/or state education agency.
4. Request assistance from ASHA's health care finance and state policy divisions.

Discussion Questions

1. How prevalent are Medicaid issues of concern to licensed ASHA certified public school clinicians?
2. How are these issues being addressed?

Background Information

American Speech-Language-Hearing Association. (1994). Medicaid issues for public school practitioners. *Asha, 36*(8), 31–32.
American Speech-Language-Hearing Association. (1994). Representation of services for insurance reimbursement or funding. *Asha, 36*(Suppl. 13), 9–10.
American Speech-Language-Hearing Association. (1991). Utilization of Medicaid and other third party funds for covered services in the schools. *Asha, 13*(Suppl. 5), 51–58.

MISLEADING THE PUBLIC

A speech-language pathologist in private practice is devoted to the utilization of oromyofunctional therapy, regardless of a client's problem. Orthodontists compose a major referral source for the practice. Children undergoing orthodontia and having swallowing patterns felt to be counterproductive to orthodontic treatment are evaluated and treated by the speech-language pathologist. Parents are required to sign a contract for a given number of sessions with a sizable amount payable prior to treatment. The fee schedule is exorbitant in relationship to fees charged by other area speech-language pathologists. Parents seeking second opinions from other speech-language pathologists regularly report that when they indicate that they do not have the funds and/or transportation to immediately enroll their child, the speech-language pathologist tells them that they are shirking their responsibility as parents and that the consequences of delayed intervention may be very serious to the child's future.

Areas of ASHA's Code of Ethics That May Apply

Principle of Ethics I, Rules A, D, E, and J
Principle of Ethics III, Rules C, D, and E
Principle of Ethics IV, Rule B

Possible Solutions

1. Inform ASHA's Ethical Practice Board and the state licensure board about the speech-language pathologist's practices.
2. Provide objective information to parents inquiring about oromyofunctional therapy.
3. Document parents' reports about these practices.

Discussion Questions

1. Would it matter if the speech-language pathologist is fully credentialed? If so, why might the speech-language pathologist be using oromyofunctional therapy procedures to treat the majority of patients regardless of problem(s)?
2. Is it ethical to demand payment up front? Does it matter if these fees compare with fees charged by other area speech-language pathologists?
3. Should clients be required to sign a contract for a given number of sessions?
4. Are parents being given accurate information about severity of the problem?
5. Is this speech-language pathologist competent?
6. Will this speech-language pathologist's practices affect the reputation of speech-language pathology in the community?
7. How might a licensure board deal with this type of situation?

Background Information

American Speech-Language-Hearing Association. (1993). Orofacial myofunctional treatment. *Asha, 35*(Suppl. 3), 91–92.
American Speech-Language-Hearing Association. (1991). Role of the speech-language pathologist in assessment and management of oral myofunctional disorders. *Asha, 33*(Suppl. 5), 7.

MISTAKEN DIAGNOSIS OF HEARING IMPAIRMENT

A child with normal hearing has been identified by another professional as being hearing impaired. Consequently, the family is receiving a monthly disability subsidy. The child has hearing aids purchased through Medicaid, but refuses to use them. The child's mother insists that the child, indeed, has a hearing impairment.

Areas of ASHA's Code of Ethics That May Apply

Principle of Ethics I, Rules A, B, D, and I
Principle of Ethics IV, Rule E

Areas of AAA's Code of Ethics That May Apply

Principle 3, rule 3a
Principle 4, Rule 4c
Principle 5, Rule 5b
Principle 8, Rule 8b

Possible Solutions

1. Arrange for a third opinion hearing evaluation.
2. Stay out of it.
3. Report the situation to Social Security Administration, Disability Determinations Unit.
4. Inform the mother of the dangers of amplification use in the presence of normal hearing.
5. Insist on an ABR evaluation.

Discussion Questions

1. Do you have an obligation to protect another professional who may have made a mistake?
2. Do you violate confidentiality when you provide an unauthorized report to an outside agency?
3. Can amplification be harmful to a person with normal hearing?

Background Information

U. S. Department of Health and Human Services, Social Security Administration. (1992). Disability evaluation under Social Security (pp. 84–85). Publication No. 64-039.

U. S. Department of Health and Human Services, Social Security Administration. (1993). Childhood disability under the Social Security Administration's Supplemental Security Income Program. Publication No. 64–048, ICN 5\436930.

Based on material from: "Interrelationship of ethics, malpractice and licensure" by G. M. Waguespack, 1995 April, Presentation at the meeting of the American Academy of Audiology, Dallas.

NEGATIVE PROGNOSIS

You are a speech-language pathologist at a long-term acute care facility. Several of the clients receiving speech-language services have progressive dementia.

Areas of ASHA's Code of Ethics That May Apply

Principle of Ethics I, Rule E

Possible Solutions

1. Discuss problems associated with accepting persons for treatment when benefit cannot reasonably be expected and continuing treatment appears unnecessary.
2. Terminate treatment.
3. Review criteria for documenting the need for services and evaluating effectiveness of treatment.

Discussion Questions

1. How can the results of speech-language services be documented?
2. How should this issue be handled by speech-language pathologists in private practice?
3. How should this issue be handled by speech-language pathologists employed by a service delivery corporation?
4. How can this problem be avoided?
5. Is it likely that such services would be delivered if funding was not available?

Background Information

American Speech-Language-Hearing Association. (1994). The protection of rights of people receiving audiology or speech-language pathology services. *Asha, 36*(1), 60–63.

Benjamin, B. J. (1995). Validation therapy: An intervention for disoriented patients with Alzheimer's disease. *Topics in Language Disorders, 15*(2), 66–74.

Clark, L. W. (1995). Interventions for persons with Alzheimer's disease: Strategies for maintaining and enhancing communicative success. *Topics in Language Disorders, 15*(2), 47–65.

Dworkin, J. P., & Hartman, D. E. (1988). *Cases in neurogenic communicative disorders*. Boston: Little, Brown, and Company.

Glickstein, J. K. (1988). *A program of functional communication skills for activities of daily living: Therapeutic intervention in Alzheimer's disease*. Rockville, MD: Aspen Publications.

Hegde, M. N., & Davis, D. (1995). *Clinical methods and practicum in speech-language pathology*. San Diego: Singular Publishing Group. Treatment efficacy, pp. 64–65.

Helm-Estabrooks, N., & Aten, J. L. (1989). *Difficult diagnoses in adult communicative disorders*. Boston: Little, Brown and Company.

Knight, R. G. (1992). *The neuropsychology of degenerative brain diseases*. Hillsdale, NJ: Lawrence Erlbaum Associates, Publishers.

Lubinski, R., & Frattali, C. (1993). Nursing home reform: The resident assessment instrument. *Asha, 35*(1), 59–62.

NEGLIGENT CLINICAL FELLOWSHIP SUPERVISOR

Your clinical fellowship supervisor does not submit the required report at the completion of the clinical fellowship.

Areas of ASHA's Code of Ethics That May Apply

Principle of Ethics IV

Possible Solutions

1. Report situation to CFY supervisor's immediate supervisor.
2. Determine if there are extenuating circumstances.
3. Determine if the supervisor had appropriate forms and instructions for reporting the completion of a clinical fellowship experience.

Discussion Questions

1. Why might the required report not have been filed?
2. Is this the supervisor's first CFY?
3. What is the worst possible outcome of this situation?

Background Information

American Speech-Language-Hearing Association. (1994). *American Speech-Language-Hearing Association membership and certification handbook.* Rockville, MD: Author.

American Speech-Language-Hearing Association. (1994). Clinical fellowship supervisor's responsibilities. *Asha, 36*(Suppl. 13), 22–23.

Crichton, L. J., & Oratio, A. R. (1984). Retrospective survey: Speech-language pathologists' clinical fellowship training. *Asha, 27*(4), 39–42.

NONCOMPLIANCE WITH IEP

A school district has difficulty recruiting enough speech-language pathologists to serve the children in the district. There are not enough speech-language pathologists in the district to provide services specified in the current individualized education plans (IEPs) for students with disabilities.

Areas of ASHA's Code of Ethics That May Apply

Principle of Ethics I, Rule B

Possible Solutions

1. Contract with speech-language pathologists from private practice to provide services until additional staff can be recruited.
2. Develop a vigorous recruitment plan in an effort to hire additional speech-language pathologists.
3. Review with administrators the mandates of IEPs in effect and the level of noncompliance caused by the staff shortage.
4. Review the legal and ethical issues involved.

Discussion Questions

1. Is the district making an honest effort to recruit additional speech-language pathologists?

2. What if speech-language pathologists are available in the community who are willing to contract their services? What if they are not available or are unwilling?
3. Is the district placed at risk by noncompliance with IEPs?
4. Are the speech-language pathologists currently employed by the district ultimately held responsible for noncompliance with IEPs?

Background Information

Failey, R. S. (1995). The individual education plan. In A. B. DeFeo (Ed.), *Parent articles 2* (pp. 205–206). Tucson, AZ: Communication Skill Builders.

Nelson, N. W. (1988). *Planning individualized speech and language intervention programs*. Tucson, AZ: Communication Skill Builders.

Wilson, C. C., Lanza, J. R., & Evans, J. S. (1992). *The IEP companion*. East Moline, IL: LinguiSystems.

PATIENT COMPETENCY AND DECISION MAKING

A patient is dysphagic and severely dysarthric, with unintelligible speech. On release from the hospital, he is sent home. The speech-language pathologist was not involved.

Areas of ASHA's Code of Ethics That May Apply

Principle I

Possible Solutions

1. Provision of patient information by the speech-language pathologist about the condition, risks associated with not managing dysphagia, and treatment alternatives for communication.
2. Involvement of the speech-language pathologist in determining competency and capacity for decision making by patients lacking communicative competency.

Discussion Questions

1. Should a patient's right to autonomy supersede competency to make decisions about whether to receive treatment or about treatment alternatives?

2. Should patients with progressive disease be given the opportunity to discuss future alternatives while competent to make decisions?
3. Do patients have the right to refuse treatment?
4. Should health care professionals be held responsible for a patient's decision to refuse treatment?

Background Information

Spremulli, M. (1995, February 27). Informed consent and communicative competency. *ADVANCE for Speech-Language Pathologists & Audiologists, 5*(8), 11.
Venesy, B. A. (1994). A clinician's guide to decision making capacity and ethically sound medical decisions. *American Journal of Physical Medicine and Rehabilitation, 74*(1), 41–48.

POOR TREATMENT FACILITIES

A speech-language pathologist has been ordered to move his treatment room four times in 6 months. His newly assigned room is poorly lighted, cold in winter, hot in warmer months, dirty, and is used for equipment storage.

Areas of ASHA's Code of Ethics That May Apply

Principle I, Rules B and C

Possible Solutions

1. Discuss with the program administrator the inadequacy of the new facility and the impact of the situation on the treatment process.
2. Provide documented cases in which legal action was taken based on the allegation that individuals receiving treatment in poorer facilities than others were being discriminated against.
3. Resign from the position.

Discussion

1. Why is there a tendency in some settings to give low priority to speech-language pathology facilities?

2. Whose responsibility is it to solve this problem?
3. Which has priority, the welfare of clients or harmonious relations with colleagues?
4. What can be done to make sure a treatment room is comfortable and free of hazards?

Background Information

American Speech-Language-Hearing Association. (1994). *American Speech-Language-Hearing Association Professional Services Board Standards and Accreditation Manual.* Rockville, MD: Author. Standard 7.0, Physical facilities and program environment, (pp. 18–19).

Dublinske, S. (1989). Action: School services (Still working in a broom closet?). *Language, Speech and Hearing Services in Schools, 20*(3), 335.

Peters-Johnson, C. (1990). Action: School services (Some groups still haven't come out of the closet). *Language, Speech and Hearing Services in Schools, 21*(1), 62.

Peters-Johnson, C. (1991). Action: School services (School district in violation for not providing adequate facilities for speech-language services). *Language, Speech and Hearing Services in Schools, 22*(1), 343–344.

POOR PROFESSIONAL RELATIONS

A speech-language pathologist is coordinator of an area cleft palate/craniofacial team. Clients referred to the team are told by the speech-language pathologist that he is the only one in the community with the qualifications to work with individuals with velopharyngeal incompetency. Parents are pressured to enroll their children in the speech-language pathologist's program and to remove them from the school or other program they already attend. When an area speech-language pathologist refers a client to the team, the team speech-language pathologist does not communicate findings and recommendations to the referring speech-language pathologist.

Areas of ASHA's Code of Ethics That May Apply

Principle of Ethics III, Rules A and D
Principle of Ethics IV, Rules B and D

Possible Solutions

1. Inform ASHA's Ethical Practice Board and the state licensure board about the speech-language pathologist's practices.

2. Make an appointment with this speech-language pathologist to discuss area professionals' perceptions of these practices.
3. Document each incident reported by parents of children referred to the team.
4. Discuss the speech-language pathologist's practices with other members of the cleft palate/craniofacial team.

Discussion Questions

1. Should area professionals continue to refer to the cleft palate/craniofacial team?
2. Will the speech-language pathologist's practices affect the reputation of speech-language pathology in the community?
3. How might a license board deal with this type of situation?

Background Information

American Cleft Palate-Craniofacial Association. (1993). Parameters for evaluation and treatment of patients with cleft lip/palate or other craniofacial anomalies. *Cleft Palate Craniofacial Journal, 30*(Suppl. 1), S2–S12.

POOR PROGNOSIS

A patient in a rehabilitation setting is not improving. The entire rehabilitation team agrees that the patient has a very poor prognosis. The patient's medical doctor refuses to discharge the patient and recommends further treatment.

Areas of ASHA's Code of Ethics That May Apply

> Principle of Ethics I, Rule E
> Principle of Ethics IV, Rule E

Possible Solutions

1. Call a team meeting with the referring physician to discuss the patient's progress and prognosis.
2. Discuss with the physician the ethical dilemma facing members of the team in this case.
3. Review with the physician the criteria being used to determine poor prognosis.

Discussion Questions

1. Does it matter if the physician regularly refers for services at the rehabilitation unit?
2. Would it matter if this is a regular occurrence when dealing with the physician?
3. Should there be opportunities for physicians to participate in team trainings?
4. What are the criteria for dismissal of a patient due to poor prognosis?

Background Information

American Speech-Language-Hearing Association. (1994). The protection of rights of people receiving audiology or speech-language pathology services. *Asha, 36*(1), 60–63.

Dworkin, J. P., & Hartman, D. E. (1988). *Cases in neurogenic communicative disorders*. Boston: Little, Brown, and Company.

Helm-Estabrooks, N., & Aten, J. L. (1989). *Difficult diagnoses in adult communicative disorders*. Boston: Little, Brown, and Company.

Lubinski, R., & Frattali, C. (1993). Nursing home reform: The resident assessment instrument. *Asha, 35*(1), 59–62.

PRACTICE OUTSIDE SCOPE OF COMPETENCE

A certified and licensed speech-language pathologist has never worked with an adult with a fluency disorder. When such an individual is referred, the speech-language pathologist begins "diagnostic treatment" in the hope that eventually something attempted in treatment will effectively lead to increased fluency.

Areas of ASHA's Code of Ethics That May Apply

Principle of Ethics I, Rules A and B
Principle of Ethics II, Rule B

Possible Solutions

1. Consult with a fluency specialist prior to beginning treatment.
2. Refer to a fluency specialist.
3. Enroll in continuing education activities targeting fluency diagnosis and treatment.

Discussion Questions

1. Can a certified/licensed speech-language pathologist be competent in diagnosing and managing all communication disorders?
2. Is specialty certification (i.e. certified fluency specialist) a good idea? Why or why not?
3. How much experience or training establishes competence?

Background Information

American Speech-Language-Hearing Association. (1993). Preferred practice patterns for the professions of speech-language pathology and audiology. *Asha, 35*(Suppl. 3), 67–68.

American Speech-Language-Hearing Association. (1990). A plan for special interest divisions and study sections. *Asha, 32*(2), 59–61.

PROFESSIONAL DISHARMONY

During a team conference in a hospital rehabilitation setting, two speech-language pathologists disagree about the benefits of continued treatment for a client. The speech-language pathologist who advocates continued treatment has maintained carefully documented progress notes to justify her recommendation. The other speech-language pathologist provides general and undocumented reasons for terminating treatment. The discussion becomes heated as the argument continues.

Areas of ASHA's Code of Ethics That May Apply

Principle of Ethics I, Rules E and H
Principle of Ethics IV, Rule D

Possible Solutions

1. Review hospital policy about appropriate record-keeping practices.
2. Review hospital criteria for determining management efficacy.
3. Provide a seminar about effective communication practices among interdisciplinary team members to assure quality client care.

Discussion Questions

1. What reason(s) other than that stated might motivate one of the speech-language pathologists to advocate dismissal of the client?
2. Does it matter if both speech-language pathologists work directly with the client?
3. Is it relevant if these clinicians often disagree about client care decisions?
4. If you were the program administrator, how might you handle this situation?

Background Information

Bowe, F. G. (1995). Ethics in early childhood special education. *Infants and Young Children, 7*(3), 28–37.

Purtilo, R. B. (1988). Ethical issues in team work: The context of rehabilitation. *Archives of Physical Medicine and Rehabilitation, 69*, 318–322.

Purtilo, R. B., & Meieu, R. H. (1993). Team challenges: Regulatory constraints and patient empowerment. *American Journal of Physical Medicine and Rehabilitation, 72*(5), 327–330.

PSYCHOGENIC HEARING LOSS

A young woman is being seen for a hearing aid evaluation. She was diagnosed with deafness when she was 3 years old. She attended and graduated from a school for the deaf and married a former classmate. She is well-integrated into the deaf community. Her speech intelligibility and English vocabulary are excellent in spite of the severity of her hearing loss. On careful testing normal bilateral hearing was found.

Areas of ASHA's Code of Ethics That May Apply

Principle of Ethics I, Rules B and D
Principle of Ethics IV, Rule G

Areas of AAA's Code of Ethics That May Apply

Principle 1
Principle 5, Rules 5a and 5d
Principle 8, Rule 8c

Possible Solutions

1. Disclose the normal hearing status to the person immediately.
2. Consult with family members, her physician, and a psychiatrist on the possible harm that could be inflicted on the woman's sense of identity, with a sudden new finding.
3. Fit the young woman with a mild hearing aid.
4. Turn in the audiologist who made the misdiagnosis 20 years ago.

Discussion Questions

1. Would this woman fit into the deaf subculture if it became known that she has normal hearing?
2. Will fitting a hearing aid on a woman with a psychogenic hearing loss effect her normal hearing?
3. Can the audiologist make a decision without consulting others?
4. Who should be consulted? How can confidentiality be protected?
5. Should the audiologist who made the initial misdiagnosis be turned in? Should the audiologist be informed of the situation?

Background Information

Zarrella, S. (1995). Hindsight is 20-20 for experienced audiologists. *ADVANCE for Speech-Language Pathologists & Audiologists, 5*(4), 5–6.

QUOTAS—1

HP Speech-Language Pathology Services expects its speech-language pathologists to bill for 32 units of client care a day.

Areas of ASHA's Code of Ethics That May Apply

Principle of Ethics I
Principle of Ethics III, Rule B

Possible Solutions

1. Give the services administration notice that you may be subject to sanctions such as loss of certification and/or licensure.

2. Notify ASHA's Ethical Practice Board and/or state licensure board.
3. If there are other speech-language pathologists, meet with employer as a group, explain concern about certification, licensure, ethical violations, and possible legal ramifications.

Discussion Questions

1. Is there a definition for speech-language services?
2. Would the service provide this care if funding was not available?
3. Explain why this could result in over-utilization of services.

Background Information

American Speech-Language-Hearing Association. (1994). Conflicts of professional interest. *Asha, 36*(Suppl. 13), 7–8.
Resnick, D. M. (1993). *Professional ethics for audiologists and speech-language pathologists.* San Diego: Singular Publishing Group.

QUOTAS—2

The B. J. Middlecat Corporation contracts all types of treatment services to nursing homes in a rural area. Speech-language pathologists are required to see a specific number of clients each day. Because of the distance between sites, on some days only one isolated site can be served. To meet her quota, the speech-language pathologist is directed to provide treatment to individuals who are seriously ill or in very poor health. The speech-language pathologist does not consider these clients to be good candidates for treatment.

Areas of ASHA's Code of Ethics That May Apply

Principle of Ethics I, Rules E and J
Principle of Ethics IV, Rules B and E

Possible Solutions

1. Inform the corporate directors that by engaging in this practice, a speech-language pathologist is subject to sanctions such as loss of certification and license.

2. Notify ASHA's Ethical Practice Board and/or state licensure board about the practice.
3. Discuss the problem with other speech-language pathologists working for the corporation and agree to meet as a group with corporate directors to express ethical and legal concerns.
4. Change nursing home assignments so that speech-language pathologists can serve more than one site each day.
5. Resign from the position.

Discussion Question

1. What are appropriate admission criteria for speech and language services?

Background Information

American Speech-Language-Hearing Association. (1994). Conflicts of professional interest. *Asha, 36*(Suppl. 13), 7–8.

REFUSAL TO REFER

A primary care physician refuses to refer a patient with dysphagia for a swallowing examination by a speech-language pathologist prior to beginning an oral feeding program administered by unskilled personnel. The team speech-language pathologist observes the patient coughing, choking, and showing clinical signs of aspiration during feeding.

Areas of ASHA's Code of Ethics That May Apply

Principle I

Possible Solutions

1. The speech-language pathologist speaks with the primary care physician about the patient's difficulties during oral feeding.
2. The medical director for the agency or hospital is informed about the situation.

Discussion Questions

1. Is the speech-language pathologist at-risk if involved in the feeding of this patient?
2. Is the speech-language pathologist at-risk if knowledgeable about dangers of orally feeding the patient, even though uninvolved in the feeding program?
3. Should the family be informed about risks associated with oral feeding of this patient? If so, who should inform them? What might the repercussions be?

Background Information

American Speech-Language-Hearing Association. (1993). Preferred practice patterns for the professions of speech-language pathology and audiology. *Asha, 35*(Suppl. 3).

REFUSAL TO TREAT MEDICARE/MEDICAID CLIENTS

A speech-language pathologist in private practice refuses to accept Medicare/Medicaid clients due to lack of secretarial help to process the paperwork and the long delay in receiving reimbursement.

Areas of ASHA's Code of Ethics That May Apply

Principle of Ethics I, Rule C

Possible Solutions

1. Refer clients to agencies that accept Medicare/Medicaid clients.
2. Determine if agencies that accept Medicare/Medicaid clients would like to contract the services to a speech-language pathologist in private practice. The agency would be responsible for the paperwork.

Discussion Questions

1. When a speech-language pathologist in private practice cannot afford the overhead expenses that certain clients, such as those on

Medicare/Medicaid, require, is the provider in violation of ethical practice by refusing to accept these clients?

Background Information

Silverman, F. H. (1992). *Legal-ethical considerations, restrictions, and obligations for clinicians who treat communication disorders.* Springfield, IL: Charles C. Thomas.

REPORTING CHILD ABUSE

A child regularly presents with bruises and burns. He refuses to talk about the injuries when questioned by the speech-language pathologist. The child has a severe delay in language development, but is improving with treatment that is paid for by the child's school district. The father brings the child for treatment and becomes angry if asked questions about the child's injuries. The speech-language pathologist is convinced that if the situation is reported to the appropriate agency, treatment will be terminated and the child's communication problem will become more severe. Furthermore, the speech-language pathologist is not certain that the injuries are abuse related.

Areas of ASHA's Code of Ethics That May Apply

Principle of Ethics I, Rules B and I

Possible Solutions

1. Ask the school nurse to examine the injuries.
2. Report observations to the proper authorities.
3. Do nothing.

Discussion Questions

1. Must suspected child abuse always be reported?
2. Why would a health professional be hesitant to report abuse?

Background Information

Brooks, C. M., Perry, N. W., Starr, S. D., & Teply, L. L. (1994). Child abuse and neglect reporting laws. *Behavioral Sciences and the Law, 12*(1), 49–64.

Brosig, C. L., & Kalichman, S. C. (1992). Clinicians' reporting of suspected child abuse: A review of the empirical literature. *Clinical Psychology Review, 12*(2), 155–158.

Fiesta, J. (1992). Protecting children: A public duty to report. *Nursing Management, 23*(7), 14–15, 17.

Hegde, M. N., & David, D. (1995). *Clinical methods and practicum in speech-language pathology.* San Diego: Singular Publishing Group. Reporting suspected child abuse, pp. 173–174.

Huxtable, M. (1994). Child protection: With liberty and justice for all. *Social Work, 39*(1), 60–66.

Needleman, H. L. (1994). Child abuse and neglect—recognition and reporting. *Journal of American College of Dentistry, 61*(1), 30–37.

O'Toole, A. W., O'Toole, R., Webster, S., & Lucal, B. (1993). Nurses' recognition and reporting of child abuse: A factorial study. *Deviant Behavior, 14*(4), 341–363.

Thompson, C. I., Fugere, R., & Cormier, B. M. (1993). The child abuse reporting laws: An ethical dilemma for professionals. *Canadian Journal of Psychiatry, 38*(8), 557–568.

Tite, R. (1993). How teachers define and respond to child abuse: The distinction between theoretical and reportable cases. *Child Abuse Neglect, 17*(5), 591–603.

SELF-CONSULTATION

You are a speech-language pathologist in an acute care residential facility. When you "think" about a client you are instructed to bill by adding time to the next session. For example, the client is billed four units for the next session, two units for the "thinking time," and two units for the actual session.

Areas of ASHA's Code of Ethics That May Apply

Principle of Ethics I, Rule J

Possible Solutions

1. Overlook the situation.

2. Discuss the possible adverse impact of the billing policy with the program director.
3. Report the practice to third-party payers and funding sources.

Discussion Questions

1. How can the "thinking" charge be documented? How can this charge be justified?
2. How could this practice have an adverse effect on the speech-language pathologist?
3. What should be done to prevent such a practice?
4. Should the practitioner check to see if the facility's administration supports this billing practice?

Background Information

American Speech-Language-Hearing Association. (1994). Representation of services for insurance reimbursement or funding. *Asha, 36*(Suppl. 13), 9–10.

SPEECH-LANGUAGE PATHOLOGY PRACTICE OUTSIDE THE SCOPE OF PRACTICE

A speech-language pathologist who works in a government facility has a natural inclination and interest in audiology, but is unable to obtain the required coursework and practicum to obtain dual certification because of geographic location and family responsibilities. He functions in a support personnel capacity with the audiologists employed in that facility; however, in the absence of both audiologists, this individual does complete hearing evaluations, fits and tests hearing aids, and makes earmolds.

Areas of ASHA's Code of Ethics That May Apply

Principle of Ethics I, Rule A
Principle of Ethics II, Rules A, B, and D
Principle of Ethics III, Rules A, B, and C
Principle of Ethics IV, Rule A

Areas of AAA's Code of Ethics That May Apply

Principle 2, Rules 2d, 2e, and 2f
Principle 6, Rule 6a

Principle 7, Rule 7a
Principle 8, Rule 8c

Possible Solutions

1. The speech-language pathologist ceases providing services except under supervision. Services will be limited to areas appropriate for support personnel.
2. The audiologist is reported for violating the Code of Ethics by allowing this situation to exist.
3. The speech-language pathologist fulfills the necessary requirements for dual certification.

Discussion Questions

1. If the speech-language pathologist has received adequate training from the audiologist, should he be able to perform these services when the audiologist is not there?
2. What are reasonable services for a speech-language pathologist to perform at support level with an audiologist?

Background Information

American Speech-Language-Hearing Association. (1990). Scope of practice. *Asha, 32*(Suppl. 2), 1.

American Speech-Language-Hearing Association. (1993). Preferred practice patterns for the professions of speech-language pathology and audiology. *Asha, 35*(Suppl. 3).

American Speech-Language-Hearing Association. (1994). Clinical practice by certificate holders in the profession in which they are not certified. *Asha, 36*(Suppl. 13), 11–12.

SPEECH THERAPY ASSISTANT

A supervisor with CCC-SLP credentials is the only certified person working in a small school district. The supervisor is assigned to supervise a "speech therapy assistant" whose assigned duties exceed those permissible according to the licensure act of the state. The school board is unwilling to hire additional personnel or to change the speech therapy assistant's assignment.

Areas of ASHA's Code of Ethics That May Apply

Principle of Ethics I
Principle of Ethics II, Rule D

Possible Solutions

1. The supervisor could resign.
2. The supervisor could file a complaint with the state's license board.
3. The supervisor could file a complaint with the school board.
4. The supervisor could refuse to sign the necessary paperwork to supervise the assistant.
5. The supervisor could maintain status quo and hope for the best.

Discussion Questions

1. If appropriately supervised, could this speech therapy assistant provide appropriate services?
2. What are the possible impacts on the licensed and certified supervisor, the school district, and the persons receiving services?

Background Information

American Speech-Language-Hearing Association. (1994). ASHA policy regarding support personnel. *Asha, 36*(Suppl. 13), 24.

Culatta, R., & Goldberg, S. A. (1995). *Stuttering therapy: An integrated approach to theory and practice.* Boston: Allyn and Bacon. Public schools, pp. 135–136.

SUPPORT PERSONNEL

A supervisor with CCC-SLP is the only certified speech-language pathologist working in a small community hospital. The supervisor is assigned to supervise a "speech therapy assistant," whose assigned duties exceed those acceptable by ASHA's Guidelines for Supportive Personnel. The hospital administrator is unwilling to hire additional personnel or to change the assignment for the speech therapy assistant.

Areas of ASHA's Code of Ethics That May Apply

Principle of Ethics I
Principle of Ethics II, Rule D

Possible Solutions

1. The supervisor informs the hospital administrator that she is violating the ASHA Code of Ethics and subject to sanctions from ASHA's Ethical Practice Board, including revocation of ASHA membership and certification.
2. The supervisor informs the hospital administrator that she is out of compliance with Codes of Ethics of national and state associations and the state's licensure board.
3. The supervisor resigns and seeks other professional opportunities.
4. She does nothing and "hopes for the best."
5. She informs the hospital board of directors about the situation.

Discussion Questions

1. What strategies might be effective in communicating with the hospital administrator?
2. Could this situation have an impact on the hospital's accreditation?

Background Information

American Speech-Language-Hearing Association. (1994). ASHA policy regarding support personnel. *Asha, 36*(Suppl. 13), 24.

American Speech-Language-Hearing Association. (1981). Employment and utilization of supportive personnel in audiology and speech-language pathology. *Asha, 23*(3), 165–169.

American Speech-Language-Hearing Association. (1995). Position statement: Training, credentialing, use and supervision of support personnel in speech-language pathology. *Asha, 37*(14), 21.

UNFUNDED INDEPENDENT JUDGMENT

A certified, licensed speech-language pathologist with 10 years of experience working with brain-injured clients recommends treatment for a client based on observation and testing. The client's insurance carrier disagrees with the recommendation based on the judgment that treatment would not be beneficial.

Areas of ASHA's Code of Ethics That May Apply

Principle of Ethics I, Rule E
Principle of Ethics IV, Rule E

Possible Solutions

1. The speech-language pathologist explains the recommendation based on test results and observations with a representative of the insurance carrier.
2. The speech-language pathologist files an appeal with the insurance carrier.
3. The speech-language pathologist withdraws the recommendation for treatment.
4. The speech-language pathologist seeks other sources of funding for treatment.

Discussion Questions

1. Did the speech-language pathologist use appropriate diagnostic and treatment terminology on the insurance forms?
2. What criteria can insurance carriers use to deny services?
3. Does funding ever have an impact on clinical judgment? Is this appropriate?

Background Information

American Speech-Language-Hearing Association. (1994). Representation of services for insurance reimbursement or funding. *Asha, 36*(Suppl. 13), 9–10.

UNSATISFACTORY CLINICAL FELLOW

A supervisor is supervising an individual completing the Clinical Fellowship Year. Although the clinical fellow came with strong recommendations as well as a good academic record, the clinical fellow's performance is unsatisfactory.

The supervisor has done everything possible to help the clinical fellow, but feels the fellow's clients are receiving inappropriate diagnosis and treatment services.

Areas of ASHA's Code of Ethics That May Apply

Principle of Ethics I, Rule A

Areas of AAA's Code of Ethics That May Apply

Principle 2, Rule 2d

Possible Solutions

1. Discuss all performance weaknesses with the clinical fellow.
2. Suggest ways performance can be improved.
3. Provide specific examples of performance issues and concerns.
4. Adjust the goals for the clinical fellowship experience.
5. Rate the clinical fellow's performance as unsatisfactory.
6. Provide more intensive supervision.
7. Recommend additional coursework in identified areas of weakness.
8. Provide structured learning experiences.
9. Terminate the clinical fellowship.
10. Offer support in identifying an alternate vocation for the clinical fellow.

Discussion Questions

1. What specific procedures should be implemented for unsatisfactory clinical fellows?
2. Why should facilities have established policies for dealing with unsatisfactory practicum students and clinical fellows?
3. How can high quality client care be maintained while simultaneously providing adequate clinical training to clinical fellows?

Background Information

American Speech-Language-Hearing Association. (1985). Clinical supervision position statement. *Asha, 27*(6), 57–60.

American Speech-Language-Hearing Association. (1994). *Manual for the Clinical Fellowship Skills Inventory—Speech-language pathology (CESI-SLP)*. Rockville, MD: Author.

American Speech-Language-Hearing Association. (1994). Clinical fellowship supervisor's responsibility. *Asha, 36*(Suppl. 13), 22–23.

Anderson, J. L. (1988). The supervisory process. Boston: College-Hill Press.

Crichton, L. J., & Oratio, A. R. (1984). Retrospective survey: Speech-language pathologists' clinical fellowship training. *Asha, 26*(4), 39–42.

Dowling, S. (1992). *Implementing the supervisory process: Theory and practice*. Englewood Cliffs, NJ: Prentice Hall.

Farmer, S. S. (1989). Assessment in supervision. In S. S. Farmer & J. L. Farmer, *Supervision in communication disorders* (pp. 274–312). Columbus, OH: Merrill Publishing Company.

Iserson, K. V. (1988). The supervision of physicians in training: An educational and ethical dilemma. *Medical Teacher, 10*(2), 195–201

UNTREATED HEARING LOSS IN A CHILD

A 10-year-old boy was referred by the school system for a hearing evaluation and a 65 dB hearing loss was identified bilaterally. He reported having difficulty hearing in school throughout his education years, but had not been identified and served by the school system earlier. His father has a hearing loss and does not wear a hearing aid. His father indicates that he does not need an aid to function, and his son does not need one, either. The family does not qualify for financial assistance from the state.

Areas of ASHA's Code of Ethics That May Apply

Principle of Ethics I, Rules B and I

Areas of AAA's Code of Ethics That May Apply

Principle 2, Rule 2a
Principle 3, Rule 3a

Possible Solutions

1. Meet with the family and explain the ramifications of the hearing loss educationally, socially, and vocationally.

2. Request assistance from the Social Services Division of the school system.
3. Turn the family in to Child Protection Services.
4. Seek assistance from the office of the Advocate for the Disabled.
5. Ignore the situation.

Discussion Questions

1. What if the family refuses to obtain amplification and services for their child even after you have met with them?
2. How can you document the necessity of your recommendation for the benefit of the child?
3. To whom is duty owed?
4. If you turn the family in to Child Protection Services, have you violated confidentiality?
5. Is it likely a pre-teen who has never worn amplification will resist your recommendation?

Background Information

Berg, F. S. (1992). Educational management of children who are hearing impaired. In R. H. Hull (Ed.), *Aural rehabilitation* (pp. 120–132). San Diego: Singular Publishing Group.

Kricos, P. B. (1987). Psychosocial aspects of hearing loss in children. In J. A. Alpiner & P. A. McCarthy (Eds.), *Rehabilitative audiology: Children and adults* (pp. 269–302). Baltimore: Williams & Wilkins.

Staab, W. J. (1991). *Hearing aids: A user's guide*. Phoenix, AZ: Wayne J. Staab.

CHAPTER 4

RESEARCH CASE STUDIES

Considerable attention has been given to ethical issues associated with research during the past few years. Issues included in this section are summarized in Table 4–1.

TABLE 4–1. Summary of Research Case Studies

Page	Title and Topic	Concepts and Issue
146	Duplicate Submission	Misrepresentation
148	Failure to Publish	Professional responsibility
149	Honorary Authorship	Determining authorship
150	Incomplete Authorship	Failure to include author
151	Incorrect Order of Authorship	Determining authorship order
152	Lazy Writing	Misrepresentation or incomplete representation

(continued)

TABLE 4–1. *(continued)*

Page	Title and Topic	Concepts and Issue
153	Plagiarism	Assigning credit: misrepresentation
155	Publication Review	Maintaining professional standards
156	Restricted Participation	Discrimination on basis of disability; failure to provide access
156	Revision Failure	Failure to honor responsibility; unjustified credit
157	Scientific Misconduct	Data fabrication
159	Subject Without Consent	Failure to obtain informed consent
160	Violation of Privileged Material	Confidentiality of information

DUPLICATE SUBMISSION

A speech-language pathologist is eager to publish information about a new strategy for clinical treatment. Furthermore, she is being reviewed for promotion and tenure at the university where she is employed. To accelerate the publication process, she submits the same manuscript to two different journals at the same time.

Areas of ASHA's Code of Ethics That May Apply

Principle of Ethics III, Rule E
Principle of Ethics IV, Rule D

Areas of AAA's Code of Ethics That May Apply

Principle 5
Principle 6, Rule 6b

Possible Solutions

1. Review guidelines of the American Speech-Language-Hearing Association and the American Academy of Audiology that prohibit duplicate submission to more than one journal at the same time.
2. Provide the speech-language pathologist with evidence that professionals must not submit the same manuscript to more than one journal at a time.
3. Base academic promotions and tenure on the quality and consistency of research and writing, instead of the quantity.

Discussion Questions

1. Why should duplicate submission be avoided?
2. Could duplicate submission result in duplicate publication?
3. What are the sanctions for duplicate submission or publication?
4. How can editors deal with duplicate submissions?
5. How often does duplicate submission of the same manuscript to different journals occur?
6. What safeguards do journals have to prevent duplicate submissions?
7. Does "publish or perish" encourage duplicate submissions?

Background Information

American Psychological Association. (1994). *Publication manual of the American Psychological Association.* Washington, DC: Author.

American Speech-Language-Hearing Association. (1992). The publication process: A guide for authors. *Journal of the National Student Speech Language Hearing Association, 19,* 138–142.

Anderson, M. (1992). *Impostors in the temple.* New York: Simon and Schuster.

Benditt, T. M. (1994). The research demands of teaching in modern higher education. In P. J. Markie (Ed.), *Professor's duties: Ethical issues in college teaching* (pp. 193–208). Lanham, MD: Rowman and Littlefield Publishers.

Fox, M. F. (1994). Scientific misconduct and editorial and peer review processes. *Journal of Higher Education, 65*(3), 298–309.

Helmick, J. W. (1994). Ethical issues in graduate education role of the faculty. In American Speech-Language-Hearing Association, *Ethics: Resources for professional preparation and practice* (4.1–4.6). Rockville, MD: American Speech-Language-Hearing Association.

Kupfersmid, J., & Wonderly, D. M. (1994). *An author's guide to publishing better articles in the behavioral sciences.* Brandon, VT: Clinical Psychology Publishing Co.

Schoefer, W. D. (1990). *Education without compromise.* San Francisco: Josey-Bass Publishers.

FAILURE TO PUBLISH

Two years ago you and a colleague presented a paper at a conference and then prepared a manuscript for submission to a professional journal. The manuscript, however, has not been submitted.

Areas of ASHA's Code of Ethics That May Apply

Principle of Ethics IV

Areas of AAA's Code of Ethics That May Apply

Principle 7

Possible Solutions

1. Submit the manuscript.
2. Review the manuscript and reconsider options.

Discussion Questions

1. How might the publication records of these individuals influence the outcome?
2. Are these individuals aware of their responsibility to increase knowledge within the profession and share research with colleagues?
3. What are some possible consequences of delaying submission of the manuscript?
4. Does it matter if the material is still current?

Background Information

Hegde, M. N. (1994). *Clinical research in communication disorders.* Austin, TX: PRO-ED.

Kupfersmid, J., & Wonderly, D. M. (1994). *An author's guide to publishing better articles in better journals in the behavioral sciences.* Brandon, VT: Clinical Psychology Publishing Company.

Pannbacker, M. H., & Middleton, G. F. (1994). *Introduction to clinical research in communication disorders.* San Diego: Singular Publishing Group.

Simon, C. M. (1994). Publishing materials: Getting started. *Asha, 36*(2), 42–43, 48.

HONORARY AUTHORSHIP

A university training program department head in communication sciences and disorders has an unwritten policy that she be listed as an author of all papers presented and/or published by faculty members within the department.

Areas of ASHA's Code of Ethics That May Apply

Principle of Ethics IV, Rule C

Areas of AAA's Code of Ethics That May Apply

Principle 8, Rule 8b

Possible Solutions

1. Review the policy for determining authorship.
2. Maintain a log book to document contributions to papers.
3. Just say "NO."

Discussion Questions

1. How prevalent is honorary authorship?
2. How can this practice be prevented?
3. How can authenticity of authorship be documented?

Background Information

American Speech-Language-Hearing Association. (1993). The publication process: A guide for authors. *Asha, 35*(3), 142.

American Speech-Language-Hearing Association. (1994). Ethics in research and professional practice. *Asha, 36*(Suppl. 13), 17–18.

American Psychological Association. (1994). *Publication manual of the American Psychological Association.* Washington, DC: Author.

Davenport, H. (1990, Summer). Ghosts who appear by degrees: The strange case of the phantom authors. *The Pharos*, 31–36.

Fields, K. L., & Price, A. R. (1993). Problems in research integrity arising from misconceptions about the ownership of research. *Academic Medicine, 68*(9), (Suppl.), 60–64.

Holzeman, W. L. (1988). Academic fraud. *Journal of Nursing Education, 27*, 309.

Huth, E. J. (1990). *How to write and publish papers in the medical sciences.* Baltimore: Williams and Wilkins.

INCOMPLETE AUTHORSHIP

A faculty member submits a student's research paper for publication. When the paper is published the student is not listed as an author.

Areas of ASHA's Code of Ethics That May Apply

Principle of Ethics IV, Rule C

Areas of AAA's Code of Ethics That May Apply

Principle 7, Rule 7b
Principle 8, Rule 8b

Possible Solutions

1. Review the departmental policy for determining authorship of student papers.
2. Training program director monitors authorship of research reports submitted by faculty and students.
3. Early discussion of authorship is included in the planning of the research.
4. Report the incident to the training program director.
5. Student confronts the faculty member.

Discussion Questions

1. How can incomplete authorship be prevented?

2. Why should incomplete authorship be prevented?

3. Is incomplete authorship prevalent?

4. Why is adequate credit important?

5. How could it be determined if the failure to credit was a result of carelessness or an inadvertent error?

Background Information

American Speech-Language-Hearing Association. (1993). The publication process: A guide for authors. *Asha, 35*, 142.

American Speech-Language-Hearing Association. (1994). Ethics in research and professional practice. *Asha, 36*(Suppl. 13), 17–18.

American Psychological Association. (1994). *Publication manual of the American Psychological Association.* Washington, DC: Author.

Braxton, J. (1991). The influence of graduate department quality on the sanctioning of scientific misconduct. *Journal of Higher Education, 62*, 87–108.

Fields, K. L., & Price, A. R. (1993). Problems in research integrity arising from misconceptions about the ownership of research. *Academic Medicine, 68*(9), 60–64.

Huth, E. J. (1990). *How to write and publish papers in the medical sciences.* Baltimore: Williams and Wilkins.

Resnick, D. M. (1993). *Professional ethics for audiologists and speech-language pathologists.* San Diego: Singular Publishing Group.

Siegel, H. S. (1991). Ethics in research. *Poultry Science, 70*(2), 271–276.

INCORRECT ORDER OF AUTHORSHIP

A student has devoted two semesters to a clinical research project. After having written the research report, the student is told that the supervisor must be listed as first author.

Areas of ASHA's Code of Ethics That May Apply

Principle of Ethics IV, Rule C

Areas of AAA's Code of Ethics That May Apply

Principle 7, Rule 7b

Possible Solutions

1. Disregard the situation.
2. Determine order of authorship relative to degree of contribution.

Discussion Questions

1. Why would one want to be first author?
2. How can order of authorship be determined?

Background Information

Huth, E. J. (1990). *How to write and publish papers in the medical sciences.*
Baltimore: Williams and Wilkins. Guidelines on authorship, pp. 229–232.
Risenberg, D., & Lundberg, G. (1990). The order of authorship: Who's on
first. *Journal of the American Medical Association, 264*(14), 1857.
Waltz, C., Nelson, B., & Chambers, S. (1985). Assigning publication credits.
Nursing Outlook, 33(5), 233–238.

LAZY WRITING

An audiologist submits a paper in which multiple paragraphs are taken from two sources.

Areas of ASHA's Code of Ethics That May Apply

Principle of Ethics III, Rule E
Principle of Ethics IV, Rule D

Areas of AAA's Code of Ethics That May Apply

Principle 6, Rule 6b
Principle 7, Rule 7b

Possible Solutions

1. Inform authors about consequences of lazy writing.
2. Establish policy about lazy writing.

Discussion Questions

1. What is lazy writing?
2. How does lazy writing differ from plagiarism?
3. How can lazy writing be avoided?

Background Information

Bordens, K., & Abbott, B. (1988). *Research design and methods.* Mountain View, CA: Mayfield Publishing.

PLAGIARISM

A paper consists primarily of entire sections copied from others' works.

Areas of ASHA's Code of Ethics That May Apply

Principle of Ethics III, Rule E
Principle of Ethics IV, Rule D

Areas of AAA's Code of Ethics That May Apply

Principle 6, Rule 6b
Principle 7, Rule 7b

Possible Solutions

1. Instruct authors about proper methods of citation.
2. Provide students with information about reference guides, such as those of the American Psychological Association (APA, 1994; Gelford & Walker, 1993a, 1993b).
3. Inform students about the consequences of plagiarism.
4. Review institution's Honor Code.

Discussion Questions

1. What is plagiarism?
2. How could it be determined if the plagiarism was deliberate or accidental?
3. How would this plagiarism have been discovered?
4. How can plagiarism be avoided?
5. What are the possible consequences for plagiarism?
6. Identify the difference between referencing sources for quotations and paraphrased information.
7. What is an uncredited paraphrase?
8. What behaviors are often associated with plagiarism?

Background Information

Anderson, M. S., Louis, K. S., & Earle, J. (1994). Disciplinary and departmental effects on observations of faculty and graduate student misconduct. *Journal of Higher Education, 65*(3), 331–350.

American Psychological Association. (1994). *Publication manual of the American Psychological Association.* Washington, DC: Author.

American Speech-Language-Hearing Association. (1994). Ethics in research and professional practice. *Asha, 36*(Suppl. 13), 17–18.

Armstrong, J. D. (1993). Plagiarism: What is it, whom does it affect, and how does one deal with it? *American Journal of Radiology, 161*, 479–484.

Bailar, J. C. (1995, April 21). The real threats to the integrity of science. *The Chronicle of Higher Education*, B1–B3.

Bradshaw, M. J., & Lowenstein, A. J. (1990). Perspectives on academic dishonesty. *Nurse Educator, 15*(5), 10–15.

Fox, M. F. (1994). Scientific misconduct and editorial and peer review process. *Journal of Higher Education, 65*(3), 298–309.

Gelford, H., & Walker, C. J. (1993a). *Mastering APA style: Instructor's resource guide.* Washington, DC: American Psychological Association.

Gelford, H., & Walker, C. J. (1993b). *Student's workbook and training guide.* Washington, DC: American Psychological Association.

Kupfersmid, J., & Wonderly, D. M. (1994). *An author's guide to publishing better articles in better journals in the behavioral sciences.* Brandon, VT: Clinical Psychology Publishing Co.

Price, A. R. (1994). Definition and boundaries of research misconduct: Perspectives from a federal government viewpoint. *Journal of Higher Education, 65*(3), 286–297.

Siegel, H. S. (1991). Ethics in research. *Poultry Science, 70*(2), 271–276.

Sigma Xi. (1991). *Honor in science.* Research Triangle Park, NC: Sigma Xi.

Steneck, N. H. (1994). Research universities and scientific misconduct. *Journal of Higher Education, 65*(3), 310–330.

PUBLICATION REVIEW

You have developed a program of vocal hygiene for adolescents and adults. A publisher agrees to publish the program, but requires that the manuscript be reduced by 30 pages. You believe that the usefulness of the program will be seriously compromised.

Areas of ASHA's Code of Ethics That May Apply

Principle of Ethics III, Rule E
Principle of Ethics IV, Rule D

Areas of AAA's Code of Ethics That May Apply

Principle 6, Rule 6b
Principle 7, Rule 7b

Possible Solutions

1. Withdraw the manuscript and submit it elsewhere.
2. Consider the publisher's recommendations and revise and resubmit the manuscript.
3. Do nothing, which would result in the manuscript not being published.
4. Ask an objective, critical colleague who is knowledgeable about voice to review the manuscript and the publisher's recommendations.
5. Consult with someone who is knowledgeable about the publishing process.

Discussion Questions

1. How could the writer's response to the publisher's recommendation be affected by previous publication experience?
2. What would you do in a similar situation? Why?

Background Information

American Speech-Language-Hearing Association. (1993). The publication process: A guide for authors. *Asha, 35*(3), 142.
Pannbacker, M. H., & Middleton G. F. (1994). *Introduction to clinical research in communication disorders.* San Diego: Singular Publishing Group.

RESTRICTED PARTICIPATION

You are nonambulatory and use an electric scooter. At your state association meeting, you are scheduled to present a poster session. You find that the poster session is on a stage and not accessible to the handicapped.

Areas of ASHA's Code of Ethics That May Apply

Principle of Ethics IV, Rule F

Possible Solutions

1. Do nothing and leave.
2. Have someone else present your session.
3. Immediately notify the local arrangements committee and the program chair.
4. Contact the association president.

Discussion Questions

1. How could this situation be prevented?
2. Why might this occur less frequently now than in the past?

Background Information

Williams, J. (1992). What do you know? What do you need to know? *Asha, 34*(6), 54–61.

REVISION FAILURE

You are one of four authors of a book about voice disorders. The publisher will not accept the manuscript unless there are major revisions of the two chapters you wrote. You chose not to revise the chapters and did not respond to the other coauthors' repeated requests for these revisions. Finally, the other coauthors revise these chapters and the manuscript is accepted for publication.

Areas of ASHA's Code of Ethics That May Apply

Principle of Ethics I
Principle of Ethics IV, Rule C

Areas of AAA's Code of Ethics That May Apply

Principle 6, Rule 6b
Principle 7, Rule 7b

Possible Solutions

1. Decline credit as an author as you had failed to complete the manuscript.
2. Do nothing and accept the royalty checks.
3. Authors periodically review contributions and revise authorship as is appropriate.

Discussion Questions

1. If this person asked for a letter of recommendation, how would this situation impact your recommendation?
2. Why would the author have failed to honor the responsibility to revise the manuscript?
3. How can authorship be reviewed and adjusted.

Background Information

American Speech-Language-Hearing Association. (1993). The publication process: A guide for authors. *Asha, 35*(3), 142.
Huth, E. J. (1990). *How to write and publish papers in the medical sciences.* Baltimore: Williams and Wilkins.

SCIENTIFIC MISCONDUCT

You are a graduate student assigned to a professor as her research assistant. The professor is working on several research projects, in addition to the project with which you are assisting. You notice that she has intentionally fabricated data on one of those projects.

Areas of ASHA's Code of Ethics That May Apply

Principle IV, Rules B, D, and G

Areas of AAA's Code of Ethics That May Apply

Principle 6, 6b
Principle 7, 7b
Principle 8, 8c

Possible Solutions

1. Ask the professor about the results of the study.
2. Report the incident to the Department Chair.
3. Do nothing; pretend you know nothing about the research.
4. Report the matter to ASHA's Ethical Practice Board and/or AAA's Ethical Practice Board.

Discussion Questions

1. How might it be determined if the fabrications were intentional?
2. Could the professor be under institutional pressures to conduct numerous independent research projects?
3. How might the option for collaborative research solve this problem?
4. How do universities monitor for scientific conduct?
5. What are the federal guidelines for scientific conduct?
6. What constitutes scientific misconduct?
7. Might the professor be competing for research funding? How might this be a factor?

Background Information

Anderson, M. S., Louis, K. S., & Earle, J. (1994). Disciplinary and departmental effects of observation of faculty and graduate student misconduct. *Journal of Higher Education, 65*(3), 331–350.

Bailar, J. C. (1995, April 21). The real threats to the integrity of science. *The Chronicle of Higher Education,* B1–B3.

Braxton, J. M. (1994). Perceptions of research misconduct and an analysis of their correlates. *Journal of Higher Education, 65*(3), 351–372.

Fox, M. F., & Braxton, J. M. (1994). Misconduct and social control in science. *Journal of Higher Education, 65*(3), 242–260.

Hackett, E. J. (1994). A social control perspective on scientific misconduct. *Journal of Higher Education, 65*(3), 242–260.

SUBJECT WITHOUT CONSENT

A child is included in a research project without notification or consent by his parents.

Areas of ASHA's Code of Ethics That May Apply

Principle of Ethics I, Rule K

Areas of AAA's Code of Ethics That May Apply

Principle 3, Rule 3a

Possible Solutions

1. Review the agency's Institutional Review Board rules for conducting research.
2. Contact the family to explain the situation and seek consent.

Discussion Questions

1. Why should clients be given information about research projects and asked for consent before participating?
2. Is clinical efficacy research during management review subject to the same rules as other research?

Background Information

American Speech-language-Hearing Association. (1994). Ethics in research and professional practice. *Asha, 36*(Suppl. 13), 17–18.

Caplan, A. L. (1988, May). Informed consent and provider-patient relationships in rehabilitation medicine. *Archives of Physical Medicine and Rehabilitation, 69,* 312–317.

Darr, K. (1991). *Ethics in health services management.* Baltimore: Health Professions Press. Chapter 9, Consent, (pp. 165–177).

Silverman, F. H. (1994). *Research design and evaluation in speech-language pathology.* Englewood Cliffs, NJ: Prentice Hall. Chapter 14, Legal and ethical considerations in clinical research, pp. 272–284.

Silverman, F. H. (1992). *Legal-ethical considerations, restrictions, and oblig-ations for clinicians who treat communicative disorders*. Springfield, IL: Charles C. Thomas Publisher.

VIOLATION OF PRIVILEGED MATERIAL

Editors and reviewers should maintain confidentiality in dealing with authors; a submitted manuscript is a privileged confidential communication. Knowing of a colleague's interest in a specific area of communication disorders, a reviewer copies a manuscript being reviewed about a related topic and gives the copy to the colleague.

Areas of ASHA's Code of Ethics That May Apply

Principle of Ethics I, Rule I

Areas of AAA's Code of Ethics That May Apply

Principle 7, Rule 7a

Possible Solutions

1. Discuss the breach of confidentiality with the reviewer and/or editor.
2. Develop ethical guidelines for editorial reviewers.
3. Pretend the situation did not occur.
4. Assume the best, such as benefit from dissemination of information.
5. Dismiss the reviewer from editorial board.

Discussion Questions

1. What if the reviewer's colleague is a rival of the manuscript's author?
2. How can irresponsible editorial and reviewer practices be prevented?
3. What course of action is available to the author of this manuscript?

Background Information

Schiedermayer, D. L., & Siegler, M. (1986). Believing what you read: Responsibilities of medical authors and editors. *Archives of Internal Medicine, 140,* 2043–2044.

CHAPTER 5

RESOURCE MATERIALS ON ETHICAL ISSUES

In recent years the speech-language pathology and audiology literature on ethical issues has increased. A chronological listing of this literature and full reference information for all listings are presented in Table 5–1.

TABLE 5–1. Literature Review: Ethics in Speech-Language Pathology and Audiology

Year	Author	Topic
1970	Paden	History of ASHA code of ethics
1976	Jones	Professional ethics
1983	Silverman	Professional ethics and law
1984	Flower	Legal and ethical considerations
1985	Metz and Folkins	Protection of human subjects

(continued)

TABLE 5–1. *(continued)*

Year	Author	Topic
1986	Green	Professional ethics and standards
1990	Hill	Leadership and professional ethics
1990	Levy and Mishkin	Solutions to ethical problems
1991	Reichert and Caruso	Ethical standards associated with clinical training
1991a	Resnick	Introduction to ethics
1991b	Resnick	Jurisdiction and diversity
1991–1992	Stromberg	Legal issues in professional ethics
1992	Resnick	Business ethics
992	Silverman	Law and professional ethics; legal and ethical considerations in research.
1992–1993	Ewing	Ethics in public education
1992–1993	Thomasma	Vulnerable individuals
1992–1993	Waggoner	Teaching professional ethics
1993	Folkins and associates	Protection of animals in research
1993	Pannbacker, Lass, and Middleton	Ethics education
1993	Resnick	Professional ethics
1994	Friel-Patti	Business ethics
1994	Gonzalez and Coleman	Ethics education: case study approach
1994	Griffith	Ethical issues in graduate education: students
1994	Helmick	Ethical issues in graduate education: faculty
1994	Keane	Business ethics

TABLE 5–1. *(continued)*

Year	Author	Topic
1994	Logemann	Ethical issues in graduate education: curriculum
1994	Pannbacker, Middleton, and Lass	Ethics education
1994	Seymour	General information

REFERENCES

Ewing, B. G. (1992–1993). Ethics in public education: All we didn't learn in kindergarten and now need to know. *National Student Speech Language Hearing Association, 20*, 125–128.

Flower, R. M. (1984). *Delivery of speech-language pathology services.* Balti-more: Williams and Wilkins.

Folkins, J. W., Gorge, M. P., Luschei, E. S., Vetter, D. K., & Watson, C. S. (1993). The use of non-human animals in speech, language, and hearing research. *Asha, 35*(4), 57–65.

Friel-Patti, S. (1994). Professional ethics and the market place. *Texas Com-municologist, 19*(6), 5–6.

Gonzalez, L. S., & Coleman, R. O. (1994). Ethics education: Students prefer case study approach. *Asha, 36*(8), 47–48.

Green, W. W. (1986). Professional standards and ethics. In R. McLauchlin (Ed.), *Speech-language pathology and audiology* (pp. 135–158). New York: Grune & Stratton.

Griffith, F. A. (1994). Ethical issues in graduate education: Student speech-language pathologists and audiologists. *Ethics: Resources for professional preparation and practice* (pp. 4.7–4.13). Rockville, MD: American Speech-Language-Hearing Association.

Helmick, J. W. (1994). Ethical issues in graduate education: Role of the faculty. *Ethics: Resources for professional preparation and practice* (pp. 4.1–4.5). Rockville, MD: American Speech-Language-Hearing Association.

Hill, D. S. (1990). Leadership and professional ethics. *Ethics: A compilation of articles inspired by the May 1990 ASHA Ethics Colloquium.* Rockville, MD: American Speech-Language-Hearing Association.

Jones, S. A. (1976). Professional ethics. *National Student Speech and Hearing Association Journal, 12*, 27–31.

Keane, M. M. (1994). Business ethics. *Asha, 36*(2), 47–48.

Levy, N. I., & Mishkin, D. B. (1990). In whose best interest is it, anyway? Solutions to ethical problems caused by influences outside the professional relationship. *Ethics: A compilation of articles inspired by the May 1990 ASHA Ethics Colloquium.* Rockville, MD: American Speech-Language-Hearing Association.

Logemann, J. A. (1994). Ethical issues in graduate education: Integration into the communication sciences and disorders curriculum. In *Ethics: Re-sources for professional preparation and practice* (pp. 4.15–4.21). Rock-ville, MD: American Speech-Language-Hearing Association.

Metz, D. E., & Folkins, J. W. (1985). Protection of human subjects in speech and hearing research. *Asha, 27*(3), 25–28.

Paden, E. (1970). *A history of the American Speech and Hearing Association: 1925–1958.* Washington, DC: American Speech and Hearing Association.

Pannbacker, M. H., Lass, N. J., & Middleton, G. F. (1993, April). Ethics education in speech-language pathology and audiology training programs. *Asha, 35*(4), 53–55.

Pannbacker, M. H., Middleton, G. F., & Lass, N. J. (1994, September). Ethics education for speech-language pathologists and audiologists. *Asha, 36*(9), 40–43.

Reichert, A. M., & Caruso, A. J. (1991). Ethical standards in the university clinic: A student perspective. *National Student Speech Language Hearing Association, 18,* 137–141.

Resnick, D. M. (1991a). Issues in ethics: An introduction to ethics. *Audiology Today, 3*(6), 13–14.

Resnick, D. M. (1991b). Issues in ethics: Jurisdiction, diversity and some rules of the game. *Audiology Today, 3*(6), 12–13.

Resnick, D. M. (1992). Issues in ethics: Balancing the ethics of a profession and a business. *Audiology Today, 4*(2), 18–20.

Resnick, D. M. (1993). *Professional ethics for audiologists and speech-language pathologists.* San Diego: Singular Publishing Group.

Seymour, C. M. (1994). Ethical considerations. In R. Lubinski & C. Frattali (Eds.), *Professional issues in speech-language pathology and audiology* (pp. 61–74). San Diego: Singular Publishing Group.

Silverman, F. H. (1983). *Legal aspects of speech-language pathology and audiology.* Englewood Cliffs, NJ: Prentice Hall.

Silverman, F. H. (1992). *Legal-ethical considerations, restrictions, and obligations for clinicians who treat communicative disorders.* Springfield, IL: Charles C. Thomas Publishers.

Stromberg, C. D. (1991–1992). Key legal issues in professional ethics. *National Student Speech-Language-Hearing Association Journal, 19,* 61–72.

Thomasma, D. C. (1992–1993). The ethics of caring for vulnerable individuals. *National Student Speech Language Hearing Association Journal, 20,* 122–124.

Waggoner, K. M. (1992–1993). Teaching professional ethics. Professional ethics, a methodology for decision making: Expert systems in the class room. *National Student Speech-Language-Hearing Association Journal, 20,* 112–121.

Listed below are additional materials about ethical issues that can be used by students, clinicians, researchers, and teachers. A short description accompanies each publication.

American Medical Association. (1990). Papers from the First International Congress on Peer Review in Biomedical Publication. *Journal of the American Medical Association, 263*(10), 1317–1444. Twenty-four papers from the first conference dealing with peer review and publication.

American Medical Association. (1994). Papers from the Second International Congress on Peer Review in Biomedical Publication. *Journal of the American Medical Association, 272*(2), 91–174. Twenty-seven papers from the second congress on issues related to peer review such as quality control, statistics, bias, blind review, and scientific misconduct.

American Speech-Language-Hearing Association. (1994). *Asha, 36*(Suppl. 13), 1–27. Contains the ASHA Code of Ethics, Ethical Practice Board practices and procedures, and discussion of 15 ethical issues including conflicts of interest, supervision of student clinicians, and ethics in research and professional practice.

American Speech-Language-Hearing Association. (1994). *Ethics: Resources for professional preparation and practice.* American Speech-Language-Hearing Association, 10801 Rockville Pike, Rockville, MD 20852-3279. Contains the ASHA Code of Ethics, issues in ethics statements, ethical scenarios, sample ethics curriculum, eight articles by recognized professionals, and a bibliography, 225 pp.

American Speech-Language-Hearing Association. (1990). *Reflections on ethics: A composition of articles inspired by the May 1990 Ethics Colloquium.* American Speech-Language-Hearing Association, 10801 Rockville Pike, Rockville, MD 20852-3279. Ten papers from the ASHA Ethics Colloquium. Topics include ethics of caring for vulnerable individuals, and ethics in public education and professional engineering.

Beauchamp, T. L., & Childress, J. F. (1989). *Principles of biomedical ethics.* Oxford University Press, 200 Madison Avenue, New York, NY 10016. Reviews ethical theories and principles; 38 case studies, 470 pp.

Darr, K. (1991). *Ethics in health services management.* Health Professions Press, P. O. Box 10624, Baltimore, MD 21285-0624. Describes various moral philosophies and principles; examines administrative procedures for making ethical decisions; details administrative ethical issues common to health services organizations; analyzes biomedical ethical issues; examines emerging ethical issues related to competition and AIDS, 292 pp.

Ducharme, S. M., Jodoin, J., Konieczny, T., & Seymour, C. M. (1993). *Classroom instructional materials for teaching ethics to students.* Charlena M. Seymour, Department of Communication Disorders, 125 Arnold House, University of Massachusetts, Amhurst, MA 01003. Materials to promote discussions about ethics within classroom settings. Includes ethics survey and results and guidelines for making ethical decisions and developing ethical scenarios, 29 pp.

Garrett, T. M., Baillie, H. W., & Garrett, R. M. (1989). *Health care ethics: Principles and problems.* Prentice Hall, Englewood Cliffs, NJ 07632. This book about applied health care ethics is for professionals and consumers of health care. It provides information about principles and problems of health care ethics as well as case studies for review and analysis, 271 pp.

Guy, M. E. (1990). *Ethical decision making in everyday working situations.* Greenwood Press, 88 Post Road West, Westport, CT 06881. Seven chapters about ethical decision making including conflicts of interest and guidelines for ethical decision making, 185 pp.

Jonsen, A. R. (1990). *The new medicine and the old ethics.* Harvard University Press, Cambridge, MA. History of medical ethics, 171 pp.

Kidder, R. M. (1995). *How good people make tough choices.* William Morrow and Company, Inc., New York, NY 10019. Provides strategies for resolving ethical dilemmas of daily living, 241 pp.

Madsen, P., & Shafritz, J. M., (Eds.). (1990). *Essentials of business ethics.* Penguin Books USA Inc., 375 Hudson Street, New York, NY 10014. Thirty-one articles about business ethics including ethical treatment of employees, management ethics, corporate ethics, environmental ethics, and multinational ethics, 407 pp.

National Student Speech-Language-Hearing Association Journal, (1992–1993), 112–135. Three articles about teaching professional ethics, ethics of caring for vulnerable individuals, and ethics in public education: (1) Ewing, B. G., Ethics in public education: All we didn't learn in kindergarten and now need to know, 125–135. (2) Thomasma, D. C., The ethics of caring for vulnerable individuals, 122–124. (3) Waggoner, K. M., Teaching professional ethics: Professional ethics, a methodology for decision making: Expert systems in the classroom, 112–121.

Resnick, D. M. (1993). *Professional ethics for audiologists and speech-language pathologists*. Singular Publishing Group, Inc., 4284 41st Street, San Diego, CA 92105–1197. Describes professional ethics including ethical, moral, and legal issues, and examples of ethical issues, 180 pp.

Sigma Xi. (1991). *Honor in science*. Sigma Xi, The Scientific Research Society, P. O. Box 13975, Research Triangle Park, NC. Provides an overview on integrity in scientific research.

Silverman, F. H. (1993). *Legal-ethical considerations, restrictions, and obligations for clinicians who treat communicative disorders*. Charles C. Thomas Publisher, 2600 South First Street, Springfield, IL 62794-9265. Discussion of legal and ethical issues related to clinical practicum and research in speech-language pathology and audiology, 249 pp.

Strike, K. A., & Soltis, J. F. (1992). *The ethics of teaching*. Teachers College Press, 1234 Amsterdam Avenue, New York, NY 10027. Describes punishment and due process, intellectual freedom, equal treatment of students, and democracy, deliberation, and reflective equilibrium, also including supplemental case studies and questions, 123 pp.

GLOSSARY

Academic dishonesty: see academic misconduct.

Academic misconduct: dishonest behavior, such as lying, cheating, and plagiarism.

Billing improprieties: inaccurate billing that can result from sloppy recording or falsification of data; may be unintentional or intentional.

Burnout: physical and emotional exhaustion that includes poor self-concept, negative attitudes, and loss of empathy.

Conflict of interest: situations in which personal and/or financial considerations compromise judgment or in which the situation appears to provide the potential for judgment to be compromised.

Continuing education: training beyond formal education.

Demarketing: reducing the demand for a particular product or service.

Dilemmas: situations in which it is difficult to make a decision.

Duplicate submission: simultaneous submission of the same manuscript to more than one journal; violation of ethical conduct.

Ethical: conforming to accepted professional standards of conduct.

Ethical Practice Board (EPB): Interprets, administers, and enforces the Code of Ethics of the American Speech-Language-Hearing Association and the American Academy of Audiology.

Ethics: moral principles or values.

Fabricating data: making up data.

Faculty practice plan: arrangement for billing; collecting and distributing clinical service income to faculty for either direct service provision or supervision of graduate students.

Fraud: Intentional deceit or misrepresentation including data fabrication, data falsification, plagiarism, unethical treatment of subjects, undisclosed conflicts of interest, violation of privileged material, irresponsible authorship credit, failure to retain data, inadequate supervision of a study, sloppy recording of data, data dredging, undisclosed repetition of a study, selective reporting of findings, failure to publish, refusal to share data, inappropriate statistical tests, misleading reporting, redundant publication, fragmentary publication, inappropriate citations, and intentional sloppy manuscript.

Honorary authorship: unjustified authorship; did not make substantial contribution to work.

Incompetent: not qualified.

Incomplete authorship: failure to include those who substantially contributed to a project.

Inflated grade: grade raised above its real value.

Lazy writing: lifting paragraph after paragraph from one or more sources; however, the source of the material is properly cited. Closely related to plagiarism.

Malpractice: negligent conduct by professional causing physical and/or emotional harm to client.

Mentor: an individual with specific expertise who provides support and guidance to another individual.

Negative prognosis: unfavorable outlook for improvement; may even regress.

Overutilization: use beyond the expected level.

Patchwork plagiarism: a direct quote in which only a few single words are changed; reference(s) not cited. Less severe form of plagiarism.

Plagiarism: thievery of style, ideas, or phrases; ranging from word-for-word (exact) to patchwork (some words changed). Often related to incorrect referencing.

Privileged material: authorization to review confidential material such as an unpublished manuscript.

Publish or perish: in academia, raises, promotions, and tenure are often based on publication.

Quota: assigned number.

Redundant publication: reporting the same study more than once; same as self-plagiarism.

Sanction: penalty. Ethical Practice Board sanctions include reprimand; censure; withhold, suspend, or revoke membership; withhold, suspend, or revoke certificate(s).

Self-plagiarism: reporting the same study more than once. Same as redundant publication.

Self-referrals: practice of referring clients to one's self.

Supervisee: one who is supervised.

Support personnel: an individual who does not have the training or experience required for professional certification. Same as aide, assistant, para-professional, or technician.

Unethical: failure to conform to accepted professional standards of ethical conduct.

Unjustified authorship: authors who do not make a substantial contribution.

Wing it: without prior preparation.

APPENDIX A

ASHA ETHICS PROGRAM

1925 ASHA organized to establish scientific standards and codes of ethics (Paden, 1970).

1930 Revision of constitution and addition of section entitled "Principles of Ethics" (Paden, 1970).

1948 Established Committee on Ethical Practices (Paden, 1970).

1951 Committee on Ethical Practices proposed revision of Code of Ethics including interpretation of ethical responsibilities of ASHA members (Paden, 1970; Silverman, 1983).

1958 Issues in ethics: Honoring of contracts (ASHA, 1958).

1970 Issues in ethics: Third party payment abuses (Bangs, 1970).

1971 Ethical Practice Board established (L. O. Cannon, personal communication, February 1, 1995).

1973 Issues in ethics: Identification of ASHA members engaged in clinical practice without certification (ASHA, 1973).

1974 Issues in ethics: Advertising of members' products (ASHA, 1974a).

1974 Issues in ethics: The bogus degree (ASHA, 1974b).

1974 Issues in ethics: Listings in telephone directories (ASHA, 1974c).

1975   Issues in ethics: Ethical Practice Board's interpretation of joint committee statement on tongue thrust (ASHA, 1975).

1976   EPB interpretation of principles governing the dispensing of products to persons with communicative disorders (ASHA, 1976a).

1976   Issues in ethics: An open letter to audiologists (ASHA, 1976b).

1976   EPB operating philosophy and procedures (ASHA, 1976c).

1977   Issues in ethics: Clinical practice by members in an area in which they are not certified (ASHA, 1977).

1978   Issues of ethics: Ethical practice inquiries: State versus ASHA decision differences (1978a).

1978   Issues in ethics: Gratuities (ASHA, 1978b).

1978   Issues in ethics: Fees for clinical service provided by students (1994b).

1979   Issues in ethics: ASHA policy regarding support personnel (ASHA, 1979).

1979   Revised Code of Ethics included issues such as advertising and dispensing of products (Silverman, 1983).

1980   Issues in ethics: CFY supervisors' responsibilities (ASHA, 1980a).

1980   Issues in ethics: Drawing cases for private practice from primary place of employment (ASHA, 1980b).

1980   Issues in ethics: Nonspeech communication (ASHA, 1980c).

1981   Guidelines for employment and utilization of support personnel (ASHA, 1981a).

1981   Issues in ethics: Public statements and public announcements (ASHA, 1981b).

1981   Position statement on nonspeech communication (ASHA, 1981c).

1982   Issues in ethics: Ethics in research and professional practice (ASHA, 1982a).

1982   Issues in ethics: Foreign degrees and degrees in other disciplines (ASHA, 1982b).

1987   Practices and procedures for appeals of EPB decisions (ASHA, 1994d).

1987   Issues in ethics: Use of graduate degrees by members and certificate holders (ASHA, 1994e).

1989   Issues in ethics: Competition (ASHA, 1989a).

1989   Issues in ethics: Prescription (ASHA, 1989b).

1989   Revised Code of Ethics (Silverman, 1992).

1989   Council on Professional Ethics (COPE) (Seymour, 1994).

1990   Ethics Colloquium (ASHA, 1990).

1991   Issues in ethics: Clinical practice by certificate holders in the profession in which they are not certified (ASHA, 1991a).

1991   Issues in ethics: Supervision of student clinicians (ASHA, 1991b).

1992   Issues in ethics: Representation of services for insurance reimbursement or funding (ASHA, 1992b).

1992   Twenty-one-page Issues in ethics Asha supplement published (ASHA, 1992a).

1993   Issues in ethics: Conflicts of professional interest (1994c).

1994   Revised Code of Ethics (ASHA, 1994f).

1994   Twenty-seven-page Issues in ethics supplement published (ASHA, 1994g).

1994   COPE developed an Issues in Ethics Statement on Subtle Forms of Discrimination (ASHA, 1994a).

REFERENCES

American Speech and Hearing Association. (1958). Issues in ethical practice: Responsibilities concerning the honoring of a verbal or written contract. *Journal of Speech and Hearing Disorders, 23,* 160–161.

American Speech and Hearing Association. (1973). Issues in ethics: Identification of members engaged in clinical practice without certification. *Asha, 15*(7), 381.

American Speech and Hearing Association. (1974a). Issues in ethics: Advertising of members' products. *Asha, 16*(1), 44.

American Speech and Hearing Association. (1974b). Issues in ethics: The bogus degree. *Asha, 16*(4), 212.

American Speech and Hearing Association. (1974c). Issues in Ethics: Guidelines for telephone directories. *Asha, 16*(11), 708–709.

American Speech and Hearing Association. (1975). EPB interpretation of "Joint Committee Statement on Tongue Thrust." *Asha, 17*(5), 331.

American Speech and Hearing Association. (1976a). Ethical practice board interpretations of principles governing the dispensing of products to persons with communicative disorders. *Asha, 18*(4), 237–240.

American Speech and Hearing Association. (1976b). Issues in ethics: An open letter to audiologists: Hearing aids and dispensing service charges. *Asha, 18*(12), 854–855.

American Speech and Hearing Association. (1976c). EPB: Operating philosophy and procedures. *Asha, 18*(8), 536–538.

American Speech and Hearing Association. (1977). Issues in ethics: Clinical practice by members in the area in which they are not certified. *Asha, 19*(5), 343.

American Speech and Hearing Association. (1978a). Issues in ethics: Ethical practice inquiries: State versus ASHA decision differences. *Asha, 20*(6), 505–506.

American Speech and Hearing Association. (1978b). Issues in ethics: Gratuities. *Asha, 20*(4), 311–312.

American Speech and Hearing Association. (1979). Issues in ethics: ASHA policies regarding supportive personnel. *Asha, 21*(6), 419.

American Speech and Hearing Association. (1980a). Issues in ethics: CFY supervisors' responsibilities. *Asha, 22*(4), 273–274.

American Speech and Hearing Association. (1980b). Issues in ethics: Drawing cases for private practice from primary place of employment. *Asha, 22*(11), 939.

American Speech and Hearing Association. (1980c). Non-speech communication: A position paper. *Asha, 22*(4), 267–272.

American Speech and Hearing Association. (1981a). Guidelines for employment and utilization of support personnel. *Asha, 23*(3), 165–169.

American Speech and Hearing Association. (1981b). Issues in ethics: Public statements and public announcements. *Asha, 23*(2), 107.

American Speech and Hearing Association. (1981c). Position statement on non-speech communication. *Asha, 23*(8), 577–591.

American Speech and Hearing Association. (1982a). Issues in ethics: Ethics in research and professional practice. *Asha, 24*(12), 1029–1031.

American Speech and Hearing Association. (1982b). Issues in ethics: Foreign degrees and degrees in other disciplines. *Asha, 24*(12), 1029.

American Speech and Hearing Association. (1989a). Issues in ethics: Competition. *Asha, 31*(9), 45.

American Speech and Hearing Association. (1989b). Issues in ethics: Prescription. *Asha, 31*(9), 45.

American Speech and Hearing Association. (1990). *Reflections on ethics: A compilation of articles inspired by the May 1990 Ethics Colloquium.* Rockville, MD: American Speech-Language-Hearing Association.

American Speech and Hearing Association. (1991a). Clinical practice by certificate holders in the profession in which they are not certified. *Asha, 33*(12), 51.

American Speech and Hearing Association. (1991b). Issues in ethics: Supervision of student clinicians. *Asha, 33*(6), 53.

American Speech and Hearing Association. (1992a). Issues in ethics. *Asha, 34*(March, Suppl. 3).

American Speech and Hearing Association. (1992b). Representation of services for insurance reimbursement or funding. *Asha, 34*(12), 73–74.

American Speech-Language-Hearing Association. (1994a). *Committee on committees: Annual report.* Rockville, MD: Author.

American Speech-Language-Hearing Association. (1994b). Fees for services provided by students. *Asha, 36*(Suppl. 13), 26.

American Speech-Language-Hearing Association. (1994c). Issues in ethics: Conflicts of professional interest. *Asha, 36*(Suppl. 13), 7–8.

American Speech-Language-Hearing Association. (1994d). Practices and procedures for appeals of EPB decisions. *Asha, 36*(Suppl. 13), 6.

American Speech-Language-Hearing Association. (1994e). Use of graduate degrees by members and certificate holders. *Asha, 36*(Suppl. 13), 16.

American Speech-Language-Hearing Association. (1994f). Code of ethics. *Asha, 36*(Suppl. 13), 1–2.

American Speech-Language-Hearing Association. (1994g). Issues in ethics. *Asha, 36*(Suppl. 13).

Bangs, J. L. (1970). Third party payment abuses. *Asha, 12*(9), 418.

Paden, E. (1970). *A history of the American Speech and Hearing Association: 1925–1958.* Washington, DC: American Speech and Hearing Association.

Seymour, C. M. (1994). Ethical considerations. In R. Lubinski & C. Frattali, (Eds), *Professional issues in speech-language pathology and audiology: A textbook* (pp. 61–74). San Diego: Singular Publishing Group.

Silverman, F. H. (1983). *Legal aspects of speech-language pathology and audiology.* Englewood Cliffs, NJ: Prentice Hall.

Silverman, F. H. (1992). *Legal-ethical considerations, restrictions, and obligations for clinicians who treat communicative disorders.* Springfield, IL: Charles C. Thomas.

A P P E N D I X   B

AAA ETHICS PROGRAM

1991   AAA publishes Code of Ethics (AAA, 1991).

1991   Issues in ethics: An introduction to ethics (Resnick, 1991a).

1991   Issues in ethics: Jurisdiction, diversity and some rules of the game (Resnick, 1991b).

1991   Point: Counterpoint: Response to Resnick's Issues in ethics: An introduction to ethics (Curran & Harford, 1991).

1992   Issues in ethics: Balancing the ethics of a profession and a business (Resnick, 1992a).

1992   Issues in ethics: Ethics and good friends are similar (Resnick, 1992b).

1994   Republication of code of ethics in Membership Directory (AAA, 1994–1995).

REFERENCES

American Academy of Audiology. (1991). Code of ethics. *Audiology Today, 3*(1), 14–16.

American Academy of Audiology. (1994–1995). Code of ethics. *American Academy of Audiology Membership Directory*, 165–169.

Curran, J. & Harford, E. (1991). Point: Counterpoint. *Audiology Today, 3*(6), 14–16.

Resnick, D. M. (1991a). Issues in ethics: An introduction to ethics. *Audiology Today, 3*(5), 13–14.

Resnick, D. M. (1991b). Issues in ethics: Jurisdiction, diversity and some rules of the game. *Audiology Today, 3*(6), 12–13.

Resnick, D. M. (1992a). Issues in ethics: Balancing the ethics of a profession and a business. *Audiology Today, 4*(2), 18–20.

Resnick, D. M. (1992b). Issues in ethics: Ethics and good friends are similar. *Audiology Today, 4*(3), 12–13.

A P P E N D I X C

CODE OF ETHICS
REVISED JANUARY 1, 1994
AMERICAN SPEECH-LANGUAGE-HEARING ASSOCIATION

Preamble

The preservation of the highest standards of integrity and ethical principles is vital to the responsible discharge of obligations in the professions of speech-language pathology and audiology. This Code of Ethics sets forth the fundamental principles and rules considered essential to this purpose.

Every individual who is (a) a member of the American Speech-Language-Hearing Association, whether certified or not, (b) a nonmember holding the Certificate of Clinical Competence from the Association, (c) an applicant for membership or certification, or (d) a Clinical Fellow seeking to fulfill standards for certification shall abide by this Code of Ethics.

Any action that violates the spirit and purpose of this Code shall be considered unethical. Failure to specify any particular responsibility or practice in this Code of Ethics shall not be construed as denial of the existence of such responsibilities or practices.

The fundamentals of ethical conduct are described by Principles of Ethics and by Rules of Ethics as they relate to responsibility to persons served, to the public, and to the professions of speech-language pathology and audiology.

Principles of Ethics, aspirational and inspirational in nature, form the underlying moral basis for the Code of Ethics. Individuals shall observe these principles as affirmative obligations under all conditions of professional activity.

Rules of Ethics are specific statements of minimally acceptable professional conduct or of prohibitions and are applicable to all individuals.

Principle of Ethics I

Individuals shall honor their responsibility to hold paramount the welfare of persons they serve professionally.

Rules of Ethics

A. Individuals shall provide all services competently.
B. Individuals shall use every resource, including referral when appropriate, to ensure that high-quality service is provided.
C. Individuals shall not discriminate in the delivery of professional services on the basis of race or ethnicity, gender, age, religion, national origin, sexual orientation, or disability.
D. Individuals shall fully inform the persons they serve of the nature and possible effects of services rendered and products dispensed.
E. Individuals shall evaluate the effectiveness of services rendered and of products dispensed and shall provide services or dispense products only when benefit can reasonably be expected.
F. Individuals shall not guarantee the results of any treatment or procedure, directly or by implication; however, they may make a reasonable statement of prognosis.
G. Individuals shall not evaluate or treat speech, language, or hearing disorders solely by correspondence.
H. Individuals shall maintain adequate records of professional services rendered and products dispensed and shall allow access to these records when appropriately authorized.
I. Individuals shall not reveal, without authorization, any professional or personal information about the person served professionally, unless required by law to do so, or unless doing so is necessary to protect the welfare of the person or of the community.
J. Individuals shall not charge for services not rendered, nor shall they misrepresent,[1] in any fash-

---

[1]For purposes of this Code of Ethics, misrepresentation includes any untrue statements or statements that are likely to mislead. Misrepresentation also includes the failure to state any information that is material and that ought, in fairness, to be considered.

ion, services rendered or products dispensed.

K. Individuals shall use persons in research or as subjects of teaching demonstrations only with their informed consent.

L. Individuals whose professional services are adversely affected by substance abuse or other health-related conditions shall seek professional assistance and, where appropriate, withdraw from the affected areas of practice.

Principle of Ethics II

Individuals shall honor their responsibility to achieve and maintain the highest level of professional competence.

Rules of Ethics

A. Individuals shall engage in the provision of clinical services only when they hold the appropriate Certificate of Clinical Competence or when they are in the certification process and are supervised by an individual who holds the appropriate Certificate of Clinical Competence.

B. Individuals shall engage in only those aspects of the professions that are within the scope of their competence, considering their level of education, training, and experience.

C. Individuals shall continue their professional development throughout their careers.

D. Individuals shall delegate the provision of clinical services only

to persons who are certified or to persons in the education or certification process who are appropriately supervised. The provision of support services may be delegated to persons who are neither certified nor in the certification process only when a certificate holder provides appropriate supervision.

E. Individuals shall prohibit any of their professional staff from providing services that exceed the staff member's competence, considering the staff member's level of education, training and experience.

F. Individuals shall ensure that all equipment used in the provision of services is in proper working order and is properly calibrated.

Principle of Ethics III

Individuals shall honor their responsibility to the public by promoting public understanding of the professions, by supporting the development of services designed to fulfill the unmet needs of the public, and by providing accurate information in all communications involving any aspect of the professions.

Rules of Ethics

A. Individuals shall not misrepresent their credentials, competence, education, training, or experience.

B. Individuals shall not participate in professional activities that constitute a conflict of interest.

C. Individuals shall not misrepresent diagnostic information, services rendered, or products dispensed or engage in any scheme or artifice to defraud in connection with obtaining payment or reimbursement for such services or products.

D. Individuals' statements to the public shall provide accurate information about the nature and management of communication disorders, about the professions, and about professional services.

E. Individuals' statements to the public—advertising, announcing, and marketing their professional services, reporting research results, and promoting products—shall adhere to prevailing professional standards and shall not contain misrepresentations.

Principle of Ethics IV

Individuals shall honor their responsibilities to the professions and their relationships with colleagues, students, and members of allied professions. Individuals shall uphold the dignity and autonomy of the professions, maintain harmonious interprofessional and intraprofessional relationships, and accept the professions' self-imposed standards.

Rules of Ethics

A. Individuals shall prohibit anyone under their supervision from engaging in any practice that violates the Code of Ethics.

B. Individuals shall not engage in dishonesty, fraud, deceit, misrepresentation, or any form of conduct that adversely reflects on the professions or on the individual's fitness to serve persons professionally.

C. Individuals shall assign credit only to those who have contributed to a publication, presentation, or product. Credit shall be assigned in proportion to the contribution and only with the contributor's consent.

D. Individuals' statements to colleagues about professional services, research results, and products shall adhere to prevailing professional standards and shall contain no misrepresentations.

E. Individuals shall not provide professional services without exercising independent professional judgment, regardless of referral source or prescription.

F. Individuals shall not discriminate in their relationships with colleagues, students, and members of allied professions on the basis of race or ethnicity, gender, age, religion, national origin, sexual orientation, or disability.

G. Individuals who have reason to believe that the Code of Ethics has been violated shall inform the Ethical Practice Board.

H. Individuals shall cooperate fully with the Ethical Practice Board in its investigation and adjudication of matters related to this Code of Ethics.

Source: American Speech-Language-Hearing Association. (1994). Code of ethics. *Asha, 36*(Suppl. 13). 1–2.

A P P E N D I X   D

CODE OF ETHICS AMERICAN ACADEMY OF AUDIOLOGY

The Code of Ethics of the American Academy of Audiology specifies professional standards that allow for the proper discharge of audiologists' responsibilities to those served, and that protect the integrity of the profession. The Code of Ethics consists of two parts. The first part, the Statement of Principles and Rules, presents precepts that members of the Academy agree to uphold. The second part, the Procedures, provides the process which enables enforcement of the Principles and Rules.

PART I. STATEMENT OF PRINCIPLES AND RULES

Principle 1: Members shall provide professional services with honesty and compassion, and shall respect the dignity, worth, and rights of those served.

Rule 1a: Individuals shall not limit the delivery of professional services on any basis that is unjustifiable or irrelevant to the need for the potential benefit from such services.

Principle 2: Members shall maintain high standards of professional competence in rendering services, providing only those professional services for which they are qualified by education and experience.

Rule 2a: Individuals shall use available resources, including referrals to other specialists, and shall not accept benefits or items of personal value for receiving or making referrals.

Rule 2b: Individuals shall exercise all reasonable precautions to avoid injury to persons in the delivery of professional services

Rule 2c: Individuals shall not provide services except in a professional relationship, and shall not discriminate in the provision of services to individuals on the basis of sex, race, religion, national origin, sexual orientation, or general health.

Rule 2d: Individuals shall provide appropriate supervision and assume full responsibility for services delegated to supportive personnel. Individuals shall not delegate any service requiring professional competence to unqualified persons.

Rule 2e: Individuals shall not permit personnel to engage in any practice that is a violation of the Code of Ethics.

Rule 2f: Individuals shall maintain professional competence, including participation in continuing education.

Principle 3: Members shall maintain the confidentiality of the information and records of those receiving services.

Rule 3a: Individuals shall not reveal to unauthorized persons any professional or personal information obtained from the person served professionally, unless required by law.

Principle 4: Members shall provide only services and products that are in the best interest of those served.

Rule 4a: Individuals shall not exploit persons in the delivery of professional services.

Rule 4b: Individuals shall not charge for services not rendered.

Rule 4c: Individuals shall not participate in activities that constitute a conflict of professional interest.

Rule 4d: Individuals shall not accept compensation for supervision or sponsorship beyond reimbursement of expenses.

Principle 5: Members shall provide accurate information about the nature and management of communicative disorders and about the services and products offered.

Rule 5a: Individuals shall provide persons served with the information a reasonable person would want to know about the nature and possible effects of services rendered, or products provided.

Rule 5b: Individuals may make a statement of prognosis, but shall not guarantee results, mislead, or misinform persons served.

Rule 5c: Individuals shall not carry out teaching or research activities in a manner that constitutes an invasion of privacy, or that fails to inform persons fully about the nature and possible effects of these activities, affording all persons informed free choice of participation.

Rule 5d: Individuals shall maintain documentation of professional services rendered.

Principle 6: Members shall comply with the ethical standards of the Academy with regard to public statements.

Rule 6a: Individuals shall not misrepresent their educational degrees, training, credentials, or competence. Only degrees earned from regionally accredited institutions in which training was obtained in audiology, or a directly related discipline, may be used in public statements concerning professional services.

Rule 6b: Individuals' public statements about professional services and products shall not contain representations or claims that are false, misleading, or deceptive.

Principle 7: Members shall honor their responsibilities to the public and to professional colleagues.

Rule 7a: Individuals shall not use professional or commercial affiliations in any way that would mislead or limit services to persons served professionally.

Rule 7b: Individuals shall inform colleagues and the public in a manner consistent with the highest professional standards about products and services they have developed.

Principle 8: Members shall uphold the dignity of the profession and freely accept the Academy's self-imposed standards.

Rule 8a: Individuals shall not violate these Principles and Rules, nor attempt to circumvent them.

Rule 8b: Individuals shall not engage in dishonesty or illegal conduct that adversely reflects on the profession.

Rule 8c: Individuals shall inform the Ethical Practice Board when there are reasons to believe that a member of the Academy may have violated the Code of Ethics.

Rule 8d: Individuals shall cooperate with the Ethical Practice Board in any matter related to the Code of Ethics.

PART II.
PROCEDURES FOR THE MANAGEMENT OF ALLEGED VIOLATIONS

INTRODUCTION

Members of the American Academy of Audiology are obligated to uphold the Code of Ethics of the Academy in their personal conduct and in the performance of their professional duties. To this end it is the responsibility of each Academy member to inform the Ethical Practice Board of possible Ethics Code violations. The processing of alleged violations of the Code of Ethics will follow the procedures specified below in an expeditious manner to ensure that violations of ethical conduct by members of the Academy are halted in the shortest time possible.

PROCEDURES

1. Suspected violations of the Code of Ethics should be reported in letter format giving documenta-

tion sufficient to support the alleged violation. Letters must be signed and addressed to:

Chair, Ethical Practice Board
American Academy of Audiology
1735 N. Lynn Street, Suite 950
Arlington, VA 22209-2022

2. Following receipt of the alleged violation the Board will request from the complainant a signed Waiver of Confidentiality indicating that the complainant will allow the Ethical Practice Board to disclose his/her name should this become necessary during investigation of the allegation. The Board may, under special circumstances, act in the absence of a signed Waiver of Confidentiality.

3. On receipt of the Waiver of Confidentiality signed by the complainant, or on the decision of the Board to assume the role of active complainant, the member(s) implicated will be notified by the Chair that an alleged violation of the Code of Ethics has been reported. Circumstances of the alleged violation will be described and the member(s) will be asked to respond fully to the allegation.

4. The chair may communicate with other individuals, agencies, and/or programs, for additional information as may be required for Board review. The accumulation of information will be accomplished as expeditiously as possible to minimize the time between initial notification of possible Code violation and final determination by the Ethical Practice Board.

5. All information pertaining to the allegation will be reviewed by members of the Ethical Practice Board and a finding reached regarding infractions of the Code. In cases of Code violation, the section(s) of the Code violated will be cited, and a sanction specified when the Ethical Practice Board decision is disseminated.

6. Members found to be in violation of the Code may appeal the decision of the Ethical Practice Board. The route of Appeal is by letter format through the Ethical Practice Board to the Executive Committee of the Academy. Requests for Appeal must:
   a. Be received by the Chair, Ethical Practice Board, within 30 days of the Ethical Practice Board notification of violation.
   b. State the basis for the appeal, and the reason(s) that the Ethical Practice Board decision should be changed.
   c. Not offer new documentation.

The decision of the Executive Committee regarding Appeals will be considered final.

SANCTIONS

1. **Reprimand.** The minimum level of punishment for a violation consists of a reprimand. Notification of the violation and the sanction is restricted to the member and the complainant.

2. **Cease and Desist Order.** Violator(s) may be required to sign a Cease and Desist Order which specifies the non-compliant behav-

ior and the terms of the Order. Notification of the violation and the sanction is made to the member and the complainant, and may on two-thirds vote of the Ethical Practice Board be reported in an official publication.

3. **Suspension of Membership.** Suspension of membership may range from a minimum of six (6) months to a maximum of twelve (12) months. During the period of suspension the violator may not participate in official Academy functions. Notification of the violation and the sanction is made to the member and the complainant and is reported in official publications of the Academy. Notifica-tion of the violation and the sanction may be extended to others as determined by the Ethical Practice Board. No refund of dues or assessments shall accrue to the member.

4. **Revocation of Membership.** Revocation of membership will be considered as the maximum punishment for a violation of the Code. Individuals whose membership is revoked are not entitled to a refund of dues or fees. One year following the date of membership revocation the individual may reapply for, but is not guaranteed, membership through normal channels and must meet the membership qualifications in effect at the time of application. Notification of the violation and the sanction is made to the member and the complainant and is reported in official publications of

the Academy for at least three(3) separate issues during the period of revocation. Special notification, as determined by the Ethical Practice Board, may be required in certain situations.

RECORDS

1. A Central Record Depository shall be maintained by the Ethical Practice Board which will be kept confidential and maintained with restricted access.
2. Complete records shall be maintained for a period of five years and then destroyed.
3. Confidentiality shall be maintained in all Ethical Practice Board discussions, correspondence, communication, deliberation, and records pertaining to members reviewed by the Ethical Practice Board.
4. No Ethical Practice Board member shall give access to records, act or speak independently, or on behalf of the Board, without the expressed permission of the Board members then active, to impose the sanction of the Board, or to interpret the findings of the Board in any manner which may place members of the Board, collectively or singly, at financial, professional, or personal risk.
5. A Book of Precedents shall be maintained by the Ethical Practice Board which shall form the basis for future findings of the Board.

Source: American Academy of Audiology. (1994–1995). Code of ethics. *American Academy of Audiology Membership Directory*, 165–169.

INDEX